P9-BYQ-446

THE PALEO CARDIOLOGIST

Praise for

THE PALEO CARDIOLOGIST

"I credit Dr. Wolfson for getting me back in the game. Other doctors counted me out, but Dr. Wolfson put together a natural plan to restore my heart health."
—**Channing Frye**, NBA basketball player

"*The Paleo Cardiologist* provides the informed, health conscious reader the tools he or she needs to naturally reduce their risk of cardiovascular disease and promote their overall health. The information contained in this book will not be provided to you by the vast majority of physicians. This is because nutrition and supplements are not taught in medical schools in any meaningful way. Most physicians are not up to date on the most recent research on supplements and prevention of cardiovascular disease. Dr. Wolfson is one of those rare pioneers who is willing to share with you what most physicians will not. The evidence based information in this book is on the cutting edge of natural options for treatment and prevention of cardiovascular disease. The Paleo Cardiologist offers a fresh perspective and should be read by all people looking to get to the root cause of disease and prevention and treatment without pharmaceuticals agents."
—**Mark Gordon**, MD, FACC, Cardiologist. Diplomat of the American Academy of Anti-aging Medicine.

"Dr. Wolfson has hit the nail on the head. Lifestyle medicine is our most powerful intervention and is the key to optimal health. He can help you turn that key and open the door to optimal vitality. Let him help you get back your life. I know that if you will let Dr Wolfson help you restore your health you will be forever grateful."
—**Trent G. Orfanos**, MD, FACC, Cardiologist. Board certified, internal medicine, cardiovascular diseases, integrative medicine, functional medicine, integrative holistic medicine and anti-aging medicine. Assistant clinical professor of medicine, Indiana University School of Medicine.

"The son of a top cardiologist follows his father's footstep and after years of practice awakens to the art and science of wellness. Dr. Jack Wolfson not only has a deep understanding of the self-healing power of the body, but is able to integrate all of his knowledge into a model of wellness that is powerful and can help people dramatically improve quality of life."

—**Keith Smigiel**, DC

"Most books for me are a skim through and a space holder on my shelf, but this one will remain by my side, yellowed from highlighter, and a spine stressed from photocopies for my patients. Dr. Wolfson is a colleague to all practitioners who wish to do the best for their patients, regardless of who may be offended."

—**Decker Weiss**, NMD, FASA, FFCC

"I have had the privilege of working with Dr Jack Wolfson in the area of critical care medicine. Like myself, Dr. Wolfson's passion for science and healing has caused an evolution. I look to Dr Wolfson as a leader in the field of Integrative Cardiology and much more. Dr Wolfson has been leading his patients to this wisdom for some time. The world and the environment need such a man of great integrity. This Doctor is standing by his convictions to bring you his knowledge in this must read book. He takes a very personal approach to deliver life changing information that is easy to follow."

—**Heidi Cunningham**, RN, Critical Care Nurse

"This excellent integrative cardiovascular book will change your perspective, diagnosis, prevention and treatment of heart disease. All the ingredients for reducing heart problems are simply and scientifically discussed in this book. I highly recommend it for you, your family and friends."

—**Mark C. Houston**, MD, MS, MSC, ABAARM, FACP, FAHA, FASH, FACN, FAARM. Associate Clinical Professor of Medicine at Vanderbilt University School of Medicine. Author of *What Your Doctor May Not Tell You About Hypertension and What Your Doctor May Not Tell You About Heart Disease*

"Jack Wolfson is the cardiologist you want in your corner. His take on cholesterol, grass-fed meat, sugar, nitrates, saturated fat, statin drugs and just about everything else he talks about in The Paleo Cardiologist is right on the money. Highly recommended!"

—**Jonny Bowden**, PhD, CNS, author of *The Great Cholesterol Myth* (with Steven Sinatra, MD) and *Smart Fat* (with Steven Masley, MD)

"*The Paleo Cardiologist* is a must read book, uniquely for those willing to accept the truth and responsibility for their own health. It provides a ray of hope, a hand in guidance and the wisdom of a Physician that changes lives. Einstein said, 'Nothing happens unless something moves.' This book will move you."

—**Michael J. Robb**, AAS, BA, DC

"Dr. Wolfson is truly an inspiration; a courageous and knowledgeable role model to people of all ages who are looking to change the world, even if it is one small truth at a time."

—**Victoria Broussard**, RN, BSN

THE PALEO
CARDIOLOGIST

THE NATURAL WAY
TO HEART HEALTH

JACK WOLFSON D.O., F.A.C.C.

New York

THE PALEO CARDIOLOGIST
THE NATURAL WAY TO HEART HEALTH

© 2015 Jack Wolfson.

All rights reserved. No portion of this book may be reproduced, stored in a retrieval system, or transmitted in any form or by any means—electronic, mechanical, photocopy, recording, scanning, or other—except for brief quotations in critical reviews or articles, without the prior written permission of the publisher.

Published in New York, New York, by Morgan James Publishing. Morgan James and The Entrepreneurial Publisher are trademarks of Morgan James, LLC.
www.MorganJamesPublishing.com

The Morgan James Speakers Group can bring authors to your live event. For more information or to book an event visit The Morgan James Speakers Group at www.TheMorganJamesSpeakersGroup.com.

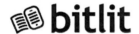

bitlit

A **free** eBook edition is available
with the purchase of this print book.

CLEARLY PRINT YOUR NAME ABOVE IN UPPER CASE

Instructions to claim your free eBook edition:
1. Download the BitLit app for Android or iOS
2. Write your name in **UPPER CASE** on the line
3. Use the BitLit app to submit a photo
4. Download your eBook to any device

ISBN 978-1-63047-580-2 paperback
ISBN 978-1-63047-581-9 eBook
Library of Congress Control Number:
2015902297

Cover Design by:
Rob Tinsman
Ave25.com

Interior Design by:
Bonnie Bushman
bonnie@caboodlegraphics.com

In an effort to support local communities and raise awareness and funds, Morgan James Publishing donates a percentage of all book sales for the life of each book to Habitat for Humanity Peninsula and Greater Williamsburg.

Get involved today, visit
www.MorganJamesBuilds.com

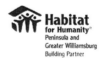

Habitat
for Humanity®
Peninsula and
Greater Williamsburg
Building Partner

Strange times are these in which we live when old and young are taught falsehoods in school. And the person who dares to tell the truth is called a lunatic and fool.
—**Plato** (427 BC)

TABLE OF CONTENTS

ACKNOWLEDGMENTS

To my children Noah and Brody: I hope this book inspires you to do what is right in the world and always follow your dreams.

To my wife and the love of my life: Heather Wolfson D.C., I owe everything to you.

A special thank you to those who shaped the person and physician I am today:

Paul Wolfson D.O., Eric Wolfson D.O., Lawrence Haspel D.O., David Braunstein D.O., Jeffrey Lakier M.D., Barbara Dudczak M.D., Nagui Sabri M.D., Leslie Brookfield M.D., Bruce Greenspahn M.D., Parag Patel D.O., Allen Rafael M.D., Mark Houston M.D., Joel Kahn M.D., Decker Weiss NMD, John Donofrio D.C., Andrew Evens D.O., and Joseph Mercola D.O.

Thank you to Marlene Wolfson, Eric and Dana Berggren, Hillary Wolfson, Jason Lubar, Dr. Paul Goodman, Sarah Dunlap, Trudi Esses, Michele Reed, Michael Reed D.C., and Joseph and Ivy Ciolli for their continuous and neverending support.

Thank you to the entire chiropractic, naturopathic, homeopathic, and natural community. We are going to change the health care system in this country.

Thank you to my editor Justin Spizman and publisher Morgan James Publishing.

PREFACE

When people ask why I wrote this book, my response is always very clear, "To change the world."

I realize this goal represents the pinnacle of ambition, but the deplorable health status in the U.S. and around the world demands leaders to wrestle control from those without our best interest at heart. Corporations and politicians for hire do not care about our health. They care about profit and power. Trillions are spent on sickness care, yet the U.S. is near the bottom of the list of developed countries in life expectancy. Those who seek a better life for us and our children must rise up, speak the truth, and vote with our wallets. Our planet is on the fast path to disaster and if we do not change course soon, we will hit a point of no return. A time where the grass no longer grows, the sun does not shine, and the oceans are empty.

The Paleo Cardiologist is your comprehensive guide to ultimate health. Not only heart health, but total body health. On the following pages, you will learn many different ways to prevent disease and stay out of the doctor's office. If you are not in control of your body, who is? The more you follow my advice, the better your health. One hundred percent dedication will lead to the best results. But any change you make will lead to a longer life, a lower risk of heart problems, and less chance of winding up with dementia or spending your final years in a nursing home. I tell many of my patients, it is okay to fall off the wagon once in a while. If you have a bad food day, wake up the following morning and have a good food day. No one can convert to a healthy lifestyle overnight. It takes time, but stay committed, and you and your family will reap the rewards of a better life.

The last ten years have been a whirlwind for me. I began my medical career as a typical cardiologist. On a daily basis, I would see dozens of patients, write dozens of prescriptions, and recommend dozens of procedures. My weekends were spent in the hospital with the sickest of the sick. Band-Aid care was given, but the revolving door in the emergency room allows the same people in over and over. The serendipitous meeting of my beautiful wife Heather put me on a path to becoming the man I am today. Now my focus is on preventing illness with nutrition, healthy lifestyle, and vitamin supplements.

Prior to writing *The Paleo Cardiologist*, I attended many conferences and read hundreds of books on health and wellness. I met with some of the greatest minds in medicine and the true pioneers of natural cures. But there is no amount of education that can replace one simple fact. It is an idea not found in any medical textbook, but is the only way to stay healthy: Stop poisoning your body and you will enjoy phenomenal health and energy. It is such common sense. Doctors spend hundreds of thousands of dollars on education over the course of many years and still are clueless about what makes us sick and what makes us healthy. They have lost common sense. The experience of opening my natural cardiology office has been nothing short of extraordinary. Those who walk through my office door are truly amazing people. Patients from all over the world seek my experience and expertise for the prevention heart disease. Others seek my opinion after suffering from a heart attack, stroke, hypertension, or heart rhythm problems. But all come to learn about the cause of their problems and find relief in the world of healthy, natural living. My patients care about themselves, their family and friends, and the world in which we all live.

My practice is so successful because I talk the talk, and walk the walk. I teach my patients about the benefits of eating organic food, free-range meat, and wild seafood. I discuss the chemicals in the environment and their impact on our health. I explain the importance of exercise and stress reduction. We do this in our house, so do it in yours. Start a garden and get backyard chickens. Tear out the carpet and put in bamboo, cork, or hardwood floors. Get rid of your toxic foam mattress and buy natural latex rubber. The world is full of people who talk about one thing, yet do another. To transform your health, and the health of those around you, you must be willing to take action. In this book, I will show you how.

The path to health is not easy and most of the world is against you. It is a major effort to stay healthy. You must dedicate time for yourself. You must make time to shop, prepare, and eat quality food. You must schedule exercise into your day. You must sleep well. If you are not healthy, your career will mean nothing. If you are not healthy, your relationships will suffer. The only person who can keep you healthy is YOU.

The following pages offer you a multitude of reasons why sickness is so common in this country and in the world. Many health books tackle only one facet of health, such as limiting sugar or getting rid of wheat. Others expose the dangers of pharmaceuticals. *The Paleo Cardiologist* teaches you about the problems of modern medicine, shows you the actual causes of disease, and puts you on a path to health. Our future doctors would be better off learning more about cause and less about covering up symptoms. For if you find the cause, you have the cure. Pharmaceuticals are not needed and expensive tests are not necessary.

This book is a game-changer. As you read and learn, your life will change. As you change your life, you will inspire others to change as well. Your children, siblings, parents, and co-workers can all learn from the lessons in this book. This is how we will change the world. If we do not speak up about what is right and what is wrong, how will things change? We can no longer sit idle while chemicals and pesticides in our air, water, and food supply are destroying the world.

Get ready to be an agent of change.

WARNING

You are about to read a very controversial book. The following information is either from medical literature or based on my years of clinical experience. My recommendations are for your information only and do not represent medical advice. Please discuss any proposed changes in your medical care or pharmaceuticals with your doctor. The opinions in this book are not in agreement with the American College of Cardiology, the American Heart Association, or any other organization with financial ties to Big Pharma and corporate America. Let the reader beware.

—**Jack Wolfson** D.O., F.A.C.C. —The Natural Cardiologist

Introduction

A LOVE STORY

For millions of years, humans thrived on this planet without disease. Their bodies grew big and strong with perfect skin and teeth. Our ancestors were full of life, energy, and vigor. Despite the need for food, shelter, and safety, stress was a small part of life. Sure, our Paleolithic ancestors contracted infections and suffered trauma, but heart disease, cancer, diabetes, and dementia did not exist. The air and water were clean. Food was everywhere with edible plants and bountiful trees. Acquiring meat required some cunning methods, but humans have used weapons for hundreds of thousands of years. Death or illness was from childbirth injury, an animal encounter, or the hard life of a warrior-like society. In most cases though, as documented by the early explorers and world navigators, Paleo people lived long, vibrant lives.

Around 10,000 years ago, people domesticated animals and grew crops such as vegetables and grain. Communities formed, eventually coalescing into towns and cities. But unfortunately, with large concentrations of people came problems with sanitation. No longer were the rivers clean because people bathed in them, as did animals. Excrement was not disposed of properly leading to pestilence, and with that came bacteria and parasites. It is here where humans sought health by using mercury, lead, and iron, all now known to be toxic. Grain was cultivated and became the main source of sustenance for many people, which is unfortunate since grains are nutrient deficient and waste vitamins and minerals, leading to many forms of disease. As humans moved to higher latitudes, vitamin D deficiency was the norm, especially during colder months. Poor intake of certain vitamins like B's and C were an unrecognized cause of illness.

Fast forward to the early 1900's in places like London, New York City, and Chicago. Sanitation was poor and clean water was limited. Tall buildings in congested cities diminished sunlight exposure, making vitamin D deficiency rampant. The importance of vegetables likely went unrecognized and fresh produce was scarce. The stockyards and slaughterhouses processed unhealthy meat. This dirty and deplorable state of affairs was well documented by Upton Sinclair in his novel, *The Jungle*. Air pollution from leaded gasoline and coal burning fireplaces created a toxic cesspool for all to breathe. All of these factors led to mass outbreaks of infections and disease from nutritional deficiency. When the population is unhealthy from malnutrition and filthy living, bacteria such as The Black Plague in the 14th century, and viruses like Influenza, can kill people in epidemic proportions. By the middle of the 20th century, urban planning improved and access to better water and food was available. Infections were no longer a major killer, so chronic health conditions emerged such as coronary blockages, hypertension, cancer, stroke, diabetes, etc. A person could survive in this environment, but not many would thrive. Disease was just a fact of life.

For my first 34 years of existence, I believed in the sickness paradigm where illness was inevitable and medical doctors came to the rescue. I was brainwashed to believe pharmaceuticals were the solution to all ailments, unless surgery was necessary to cure. I thought the government was going to take care of us with advice such as the Food Pyramid and "Milk does the body good." I trusted corporate America to create healthy foods packed with all the necessary nutrients. Born during Nixon's war on cancer and the rise of the American Heart Association (both of which are failures), I was set on becoming a doctor. My father was a cardiologist and saved lives, so with the encouragement of my mom, I followed the same path at the Chicago College of Osteopathic Medicine.

In medical school, the glories of modern medicine echoed throughout the halls. My classmates and I were eager to learn about drugs and longed to write that first prescription. Blood pressure is high? Take a pill to make it lower. Cholesterol is high? Take a pill to make it lower. We watched surgical procedures with awe, as the "useless" organ was removed and disease bypassed. We were led to believe body parts such as the gall bladder and appendix, organs we evolved with for millions of years, were useless. If an artery is blocked, open it with a balloon and it will be as good as new. Vaccination benefits were never debated, but rather just accepted as gospel to rid the world of disease. Nutrition was never discussed. Exercise got the rare mention as, like the Nike slogan, we told our patients to "Just Do It." The actual cause of disease was not a concern. During those years, words like organic and natural were not in my vocabulary. If they were used, it was only amongst quacks and kooks, tree huggers if you will. In ten years of post-graduate training, topics like nutrition, supplements, and the dangers of chemicals were never discussed. Unfortunately, I never questioned the current state of medical training. I do not have regrets. Every event on my journey had a purpose.

I had many mentors during my training, but none as important as my dad. Dr. Paul Wolfson was my role model and hero. Always the life of the party, he was full of jokes and exhilarating stories. His father was a butcher from Atlantic City, and from those beginnings my father went to osteopathic medical school, finishing first in his class. I still encounter his classmates who marvel at my dad's photographic memory. He went on to become the first D.O. resident at the prestigious Cleveland Clinic and eventually the head of Cardiology at Midwestern University. He was well published in medical journals and well respected around the world.

Strangely and abruptly, in his mid-fifties, he became depressed. Our family could not figure out why this guy who had money, prestige, health, and people who loved him, was not happy. His emotion and passion for life were gone. My dad used to be the center of attention at every event, but he was now reduced to just part of the crowd. Friends commented they wanted to "shake him" to wake him up. We took my father to a psychiatrist who was just another pill pusher and offered no help. My family and I were outright dejected.

His depression was followed by frequent falls, problems swallowing, and a lack of facial expression. Parkinsonism was the next label, and then ultimately his final diagnosis, PSP or Progressive Supranuclear Palsy. The Mayo Clinic predicted my dad would live a few more years and he lived those years in agony. His demise was cruel torture to such an incredible man. He passed away in 2007, shortly after seeing my newborn son Noah for the first and only time. My father was robbed of the opportunity to love his wife for many more years, to see his children succeed in the world and build their families, and to live a full life.

How did this happen? Was it genetic? Why couldn't the doctors at the esteemed Mayo Clinic help him? The answer to these questions arrived in the form of a young woman and a chance encounter at a farmer's market. Just prior to my 34th birthday, this girl turned my world upside down. She confidently stated that medical doctors were not actually healing anyone, just covering up problems. She professed pharmaceuticals were rarely necessary and most medical procedures were not needed. Most doctors would laugh and scoff at this person, for those opinions rattle the entire foundation of medical education. But to me her comments made sense (it also helped that she is very beautiful). For some time, I had been frustrated at all the patient illness and poor outcomes, despite the pills and procedures. My father became a vegetable and the doctors couldn't do a thing.

This incredible woman is now my wife Heather. She is a doctor of chiropractic, herself from good stock with a very intelligent mother and a father who is a chiropractor with hands that heal. I learned from Heather that poor nutrition and chemicals were the culprits of my father's demise. This epiphany of CAUSE turns out to be the reason for just about all disease, save a few rare genetic errors and birth defects. My dad enjoyed throwing back a few too many drinks, did not eat well, had a potbelly, slept poorly, and lived most of his adult life working in a hospital. Part of the job description of a cardiologist is plenty of time in the hospital performing procedures that require massive radiation exposure. Radiation damages the body and is a cause of many diseases. A hospital, with all the chemicals and infections, is the sickest, most toxic place in the world.

Watching my dad's destruction horrified me, given I was leading the same life he did. I was a cardiologist who did not eat well, liked to drink a little too much, and worked way too many hours in a toxic hospital. I was exposed to radiation daily in the catheterization lab doing pacemakers and angiograms. This all had to change, fast! I soon gave up the procedures involving radiation. I met with natural doctors like homeopaths, chiropractors, and naturopaths. I read medical journals with a more critical eye, not blindly trusting the drug rep for my information. I attended natural healthcare conferences and voraciously read any book I could find that taught wellness and the cause of disease. Authors like Gary Taubes and Rachel Carson were my new mentors.

My colleagues laughed behind my back and undermined me at every opportunity. They had no interest in learning natural remedies or the cause of disease. Doctors hate change. Doctors do not want to be questioned. Unfortunately, it is the patient who suffers. The head of the cardiology practice informed me that my new religion of health would decrease revenue and was not welcome. "Ordering studies and procedures is how you get paid Dr. Wolfson." I was forced to apologize to referring doctors for stopping their patients' pharmaceuticals and for recommending nutritional/lifestyle changes. One large referral source actually threatened to pull all their patients from our care. I was warned that revenue would be deducted from my salary. It was time to leave.

In 2012, I started my own practice, Wolfson Integrative Cardiology. The response has been tremendous. Patients from all over the world seek my consultation. I spend 1-2 hours on new patient visits and 45 minutes and more for follow-ups. I perform the most advanced blood tests to prevent disease from starting or progressing. The typical cardiologist only has the two P's at their disposal—pills and procedures. By testing for heavy metals, food sensitivities, hormones, intracellular nutrients, gut function, parasites, and so much more, I provide a plan for health recovery and life longevity. Check out the hundreds of testimonials on my website endorsing my success.

The transition to my own practice was made possible by my rock and the love of my life: I owe it all to Heather. I am an incredible father, doting husband, and custodian of the environment. Because of Heather, I transformed from a doctor who followed mindless, pharmaceutical directed, cookbook medicine to a leader of the health revolution in this country. My goal is to go after the CAUSE of disease. When you remove the CAUSE, the body will heal itself.

Writing this book was no easy task, as I love to spend every spare minute with family and friends, but the world needs to know the real reasons people develop disease and the solution to prevent it. The book starts with the most controversial topic in cardiology: cholesterol. We discuss the critical nature of cholesterol and LDL, commonly known as the bad cholesterol. Then, we dive into the importance of Paleo nutrition, the diet our ancestors enjoyed and evolved with for millions of years. Those who veer from Paleo are bound for illness. Through the eyes of a cardiologist, I guide you through which foods are healthy and which are to be avoided for optimum health. Then, I share information and education about toxins such as plastics and air pollution, and how to minimize their damage. I discuss heavy metals along with the science regarding removing them from the body. Lack of exercise, lack of sleep, and the modern stress-heavy lifestyle are trends that need to be reversed, and I walk you through how to make this happen. I also go in depth looking at the most important tests to really determine risk, and I provide data on the best supplements to consume for optimum cardiovascular prevention. Although I am a cardiologist, the principals of this book will apply to everyone. The recommendations in the following chapters will revitalize your health, no matter your symptoms or disease. If we feed our body the right nutrition, avoid chemicals, get the toxins out, and take the right supplements, this machine called the human body will repair itself.

Together, Heather and I are The Drs. Wolfson. Our goal is to make the planet a safer place for ourselves, our children, and our children's children. We are looking for people with the same passion and purpose. We are changing the world. Please, join us in the health revolution—together we will make the world a better place.

➤➤—▷ **Chapter 1** ◁—◅◅

CHOLESTEROL IS KING

"If you repeat a lie often enough, it becomes truth"
—Unknown

J ust say the word cholesterol out loud. What images does it conjure up? Perhaps a person having a heart attack or stroke, a vessel clogged with yellow plaque, or maybe a juicy cheeseburger? Your preconceived notions are all the result of an aggressive marketing campaign by pharmaceutical companies to generate fear. The scare propaganda gets you to take drugs leading to trillions of dollars in the coffers of "Big Pharma."

But ask yourself, your doctor, or even your next-door neighbor, "What is cholesterol? What does it do and why does my body make it? Why is cholesterol present in dogs, chickens, cows, and gorillas? If it is harmful, is my body trying to cause a heart attack or a stroke?" Chances are, whomever you ask, will not give you the correct answer. Your doctor is likely to give you a blank stare or quickly get intimidated, possibly kicking you out of his or her office.

These questions seem foolish because if the body is making cholesterol, there is an obvious purpose. In fact, everything the human body does is for a reason. Cholesterol is a small molecule made by all mammals that contains three different elements or atoms: carbon, hydrogen, and oxygen. This "scary" substance contains only these three basic elements. We are not talking about dangerous heavy metals like mercury and lead, or the harmful chemicals in plastic. Carbon, hydrogen, and oxygen are the building blocks of life. Cholesterol is a pretty basic structure that has been around for hundreds of millions of years. This fact was drilled into young, fertile minds during medical school, but was later suffocated by the tentacles of "Big Pharma" and their cheerleaders in the media. This chapter will dispel the unfounded negativity surrounding cholesterol and give you confidence that eating cholesterol-containing foods is critical to health.

CHOLESTEROL 101

Cholesterol is a hydrophobic, wax-like molecule, meaning it does not like water; it prefers the company of fat. Picture a pot of chicken soup left out all night, which develops a thick layer of fat on top (which you can use to fry eggs, vegetables, etc.). Because of its unique structure, cholesterol must travel around the body with "friends" called LDL and HDL (more on lipoproteins in the next chapter). A large percentage of cholesterol production occurs in the liver, an organ in the upper right portion of your abdomen. The liver is responsible for many functions including detoxification (removing the gunk from the body), the manufacturing of proteins and fats, storage and breakdown of sugar, digestion of food, and making cholesterol. The body makes about 1000 mg of cholesterol daily, enough to fill a vitamin capsule. Very low cholesterol is a bad sign the liver is not functioning and is associated with cancer risk and death.

★LIVE WELL: Keep your liver healthy by eating right and avoiding chemicals.

Cholesterol is found in all animal sources of food because animal cells contain it, just like human cells do. The typical daily consumption of cholesterol in the U.S. is 200-300 mg, about the weight of 3 raindrops. Most of the cholesterol from food is not absorbed, but preferentially passed in the stool. The gut prefers to absorb the cholesterol made by the liver and passed into the bile to assist with digestion. There are some pharmaceuticals and natural supplements, which prevent reabsorption as a way to lower cholesterol numbers. Most people either make a lot or absorb a lot, which stands to reason because of the importance of this molecule. There are tests available to determine if you are a hyper-absorber or a hyper-synthesizer of cholesterol. Of note, insulin released in response to sugar and carbohydrate ingestion stimulates the HMG-CoA reductase enzyme to produce excess cholesterol.

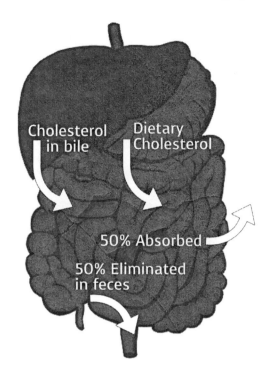

★**LIVE WELL**: Decreasing sugar intake is one of the best ways to control excess cholesterol.

So now that you understand the structure of the tiny cholesterol molecule, we can discuss why the human body and every animal on the planet produce it. The truth, encoded in our DNA, is the desire for the body to give itself a heart attack or stroke? How moronic does that sound? Our DNA and genetics are not trying to kill us. Yet this is the garbage spewed by doctors and pharmaceutical companies on a daily basis. Tens of billions of dollars wasted under the false pretense that cholesterol is harmful. Handfuls of pills, side effects galore, and lost time for blood tests and prescription refills highlight the runaway drug train. Read on to learn the critical importance of cholesterol, the "can't live without" substance.

TESTOSTERONE, ESTROGEN, PROGESTERONE

Extra! Extra! Testosterone is made from cholesterol. Got your attention now guys? Without cholesterol to make testosterone, your libido disappears and your erections are more like a wet noodle. Women also produce testosterone as part of their delicate hormone balance. Testosterone increases muscle mass and leads to improved bone density and strength. Without enough cholesterol, testosterone production has to suffer. Low "T" is linked to Alzheimer's dementia[1] and coronary artery disease.[2] In fact, it is well known testosterone supplementation reduces LDL (low-density lipoprotein). But don't run out to fill your script for testosterone just yet. The reason LDL is reduced is because the liver does not see the need to produce cholesterol for testosterone production. The body is getting it externally. The testicles cry out for cholesterol when the body wants to produce testosterone. The liver makes it and packages it up in the LDL carrier, or LDL "bus" as I call it. (More on LDL in Chapter 2). I am not saying all erectile and libido issues are related to cholesterol, but I am saying the body needs cholesterol; therefore, lowering cholesterol does not seem to be in the best interest for someone looking to increase sex hormone production.

The female sex hormones progesterone and estrogen come from—you guessed it, our friend cholesterol. Progesterone is produced in the ovaries, adrenal glands, and in the placenta during pregnancy. It is a crime for a premenopausal woman to be put on a cholesterol reducing pharmaceutical, since we have no idea if this affects fertility or fetal development. After menopause, sex-hormone production decreases and is largely responsible for symptoms. It seems to me we would want cholesterol around to form these hormones and minimize hot flashes, low libido, and a general cantankerous attitude towards unfortunate husbands (ha-ha). There is a lot of controversy regarding post-menopausal hormone prescriptions, but there should be no confusion about letting the body produce what it naturally wants without inhibition by cholesterol reducing drugs. Could a vegan diet, void of cholesterol, limit hormone production?

Finally, the most prevalent sex hormone in circulation is DHEA. This master molecule is converted into estrogen and testosterone. DHEA is made in the adrenals, testes, and ovaries from cholesterol. Hundreds of studies prove that a low DHEA level is associated with an increased risk of heart attack, stroke, diabetes, and just about everything else.[3] One scary fact is that vegan women suffer from lower DHEA levels as compared to Paleo eaters (more on Paleo in Chapter 3).[4] Whether or not DHEA supplementation is beneficial is a subject of debate. I usually recommend it when levels are found to be low through saliva or blood testing.

★**LIVE WELL**: Male and female hormones are made from cholesterol.

ENERGY

Do you constantly feel tired or fatigued? Do you need Starbucks to get through this chapter? (I hope not, since I wrote it). If you are regularly fatigued, it could be a cortisol problem. You see, cortisol is the main energy hormone of the body, and cortisol is made from cholesterol. If a tiger is chasing you, cortisol is pumped out of the adrenal glands like oil in the Gulf. Its primary functions are: to increase blood sugar (critical in times of stress); balance the immune system; and aid in fat, protein and carbohydrate metabolism. Cortisol maintains blood pressure and is important for stomach acid secretion. If the stomach does not produce enough acid, digestion is poor, and nutrients are not absorbed. The consequences are staggering. Cortisol production is markedly diminished in many people because of poor nutrition (sugar and caffeine), chemicals, lack of sleep, and chronic stress. By trying to decrease cholesterol, we are tying both hands behind the back of the adrenal gland and limiting the creation of cortisol.

Aldosterone is another vital hormone, and is responsible for salt retention in the kidneys. We are all taught salt is bad, but I assure you, we cannot live without sodium. Despite all the negative press, sodium is a precious element. Salt (or sodium) retention is responsible for blood pressure maintenance: No pressure equals no life. Guess where aldosterone comes from? Yep, our friend cholesterol.

★**LIVE WELL**: Cortisol is the energy hormone that comes from cholesterol.

Thyroid hormones T3 and T4 are responsible for temperature maintenance, cell metabolism and energy. Symptoms of low thyroid include constipation, poor sleep, dry skin, and weight gain. Theses hormones are actually made from the amino acid tyrosine and iodine, not cholesterol. I am discussing the thyroid here because the follicular cells in the thyroid responsible for hormone production all contain cholesterol (as does every cell in the body).

Are you getting the picture yet? The drug companies and their doctors on the payroll are demonizing this critical molecule, yet as discussed, cholesterol is crucial for living a healthy life. But wait, cholesterol does so much more.

Most people heard the news that vitamin D is essential for health. It builds strong bones, normalizes blood pressure, boosts immune function, and decreases the risk of cancer. How is it made? Cholesterol travels through small vessels in the skin where sunlight converts it into vitamin D. Vitamin D then requires optimal liver and kidney function to be converted to a useable form. Vitamin D is very easy to measure and I prefer my patients achieve a level higher than 50 (more in Chapter 16 about vitamin D supplementation). Some people make vitamin D but it doesn't function because of a genetic defect. Is your doctor testing you for this gene defect? They should.[5]

LET THE SUN SHINE IN

Despite the negative press, the TRUTH is the sun is critical for life. Living in northern climates increases your risk of several diseases, presumably from less sun exposure. Multiple Sclerosis (MS) is a disease that affects the myelin sheath of nerve cells in the body. This sheath is like the insulation on a wire, so when you put your hand on a hot stove, you sense it and jerk your hand away before it burns. This response relies on the speed of your nerves, which is heavily influenced by the myelin sheath. There are many symptoms of MS, but clearly, the less sun you get, the higher your risk.[6]

Getting full-body sun exposure for 15-30 minutes a day is critical for health. Our Paleo ancestors were outside all day long! Remember the phrase, "Where the sun don't shine?" Don't have an area on your body that fits that saying. Just be careful to avoid a sunburn. And remember, if our body does not make cholesterol, it cannot produce vitamin D. Our family usually runs around the backyard naked to soak up the sun. Don't be shocked if you come by for a visit.

BRAIN HEALTH

The brain has countless responsibilities such as movement, sensation, thought, memories, sight, and hearing. Did you know the brain is loaded with fat and cholesterol? A recent study found the people with the highest cholesterol levels have the best memory.[7] Another report concluded people with low cholesterol had higher rates of depression, aggression, and suicidal thoughts.[8] Over the years, I realized vegan patients do not think as clearly and suffer from more hormonal issues compared to meat eaters. Breast milk contains fat and cholesterol because those are what a baby's brain needs. Infants can live for years on breast milk alone. Would the human body secrete a deleterious substance to nurse its young? Would mammals feed their offspring with cholesterol-laden milk if it were harmful? A chicken cannot grow inside an egg without the cholesterol in the yolk.

If you do not eat animal products, you do not give your body the nutrients it needs to make cholesterol. If we lower cholesterol with pharmaceuticals, our levels are decreased everywhere in the body. Do we really want to lower cholesterol from our brain? For a great read debunking veganism, check out *The Vegetarian Myth* by Lierre Keith Ph.D.

★**LIVE WELL**: Find out if you were breast-fed and encourage all moms to do so.

DIGESTION

Another critical function using cholesterol is digestion. If we do not digest food properly, even the best foods will not be absorbed. Cholesterol is secreted by the liver into the bile ducts to help digest food. Ask someone without a gall bladder, removed in a procedure called a cholecystectomy, what happens if they eat oily or fatty foods. Usually, diarrhea is a consequence of those meals. It is because the gall bladder stores bile salts and squirts it onto fats to aid in their breakdown. Without the cholesterol and bile salts, our digestion is poor, nutrients are not absorbed, and disease is inevitable. Doctors claim the gall bladder is not necessary. Oh, how wrong they are. If a doc is recommending the removal of this organ, get a second opinion from a natural doctor ASAP.

★**LIVE WELL**: A healthy gall bladder is vitally important.

CELL MEMBRANE

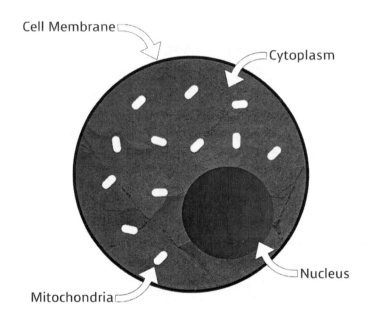

The human body is made up of trillions of cells. Each of those tiny cells is held in place by a thin layer called the cell membrane, much like a house surrounded by a fence. Cholesterol is an integral part of the cell membrane. It helps keep the fence strong yet fluid so cells can communicate with each other, keep important contents in, and keep unwanted particles out. Hormones, vitamins, minerals, and hundreds of other tiny molecules enter and exit cells based on the integrity and health of the cell membrane. Our intestines are lined with cells, which form a tight barrier, limiting what molecules come in to our body. Could one cause leading to the rise of Leaky Gut syndrome be from so many millions taking cholesterol-reducing drugs? (More on Leaky Gut in Chapter 10). One of the first organs damaged on the pathway to cardiovascular disease is the endothelium. This single layer of cells lines our blood vessels and is critical to heart health. If the endothelium does not function, the equivalent of a forest fire starts in the vessel wall with the end result of plaque creation and a possible heart attack. Communication between cells is one of the keys to life, and it is dependent on cholesterol.

★**LIVE WELL**: Every single cell in the human body contains cholesterol.

IS HIGH CHOLESTEROL ASSOCIATED WITH HEART DISEASE?

The MRFIT study, a landmark cardiovascular study undertaken in the 1970's, provided tremendous data on a large population and risk factors for heart disease. The following graph was published to demonstrate cholesterol levels and mortality (death rates) over the course of six years.

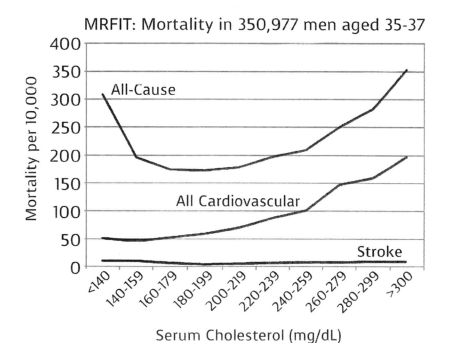

We can see in the above chart, all-cause mortality is the same from the cholesterol range of 150-250. You read that correctly. The chances of dying are the same whether your total cholesterol is 150 or 250! Notice the striking increase in all-cause mortality at the lowest levels of cholesterol (top left). I start the search for cancer in my patients with cholesterol less than 150. Finally, notice how total cholesterol has nothing to do with the chance of dying from a stroke.

Humans evolved over millions of years. Our DNA is essentially perfect, until the damage from poor nutrition and chemicals occurs. These two categories influence the way our DNA is put to use. Broccoli can trigger a gene to turn on, while pizza can turn it off. Discussing nutrition and chemicals will make up a large part of this book and is the foundation of prevention and treatment of disease.

CASE STUDY

Todd P. was a middle age male with fatigue and low total cholesterol. He was vegan for years and considered introducing meat back into his diet. Of course, I thought this was a fabulous idea. Adding meat back to the diet has to be done slowly and carefully. Many vegans complain of digestive issues when resuming animal foods. This is because the vegan body is deficient and does not have the tools needed to digest meat. It is best to start slow and use digestive enzymes to get through the early stages of any dietary change. I tested Todd's cortisol levels, which were very low. Within four months of adding meat and seafood, along with plenty of coconut oil, Todd's cholesterol went from 123 to 186. He felt great and regained all his lost energy.

ACTION PLAN

1. Cholesterol is critical to the function of every cell in the body.
2. Hormones, vitamin D, and digestive juices all come from cholesterol.
3. The cell membrane is a cholesterol-rich structure vital to health.
4. The more cholesterol in your brain, the less your risk of dementia, depression, and other neurologic diseases.
5. Eat cholesterol-rich foods. They will make you live longer.

If we were misled regarding the dangers of cholesterol, what other misinformation are corporations and the government feeding us? Are we really to believe air pollution is not a health concern and cell phones are safe? Are organic foods really a waste of money? Is five hours enough time to sleep? Is the reason humans live so long because of the massive vaccine program or the average adult swallowing more than three prescription drugs per day?

Continue reading this book to find out the problems with modern medicine and the real cure of disease . . . finding the CAUSE.

Chapter 2

LDL IS NOT
THE BOOGIE MAN

"Physicians think they are doing something for you
by labeling what you have as a disease."
—Immanuel Kant

F or years we've been told there is good cholesterol and bad cholesterol. We want lots of good and not a lot of bad. The bad cholesterol in question is known as LDL, or low-density lipoprotein. The good is HDL, or high-density lipoprotein. The truth is, both are critically important and human life would not exist without them.

LIPOPROTEINS EXPLAINED

LDL and HDL represent a class of molecules called lipoproteins. Lipoproteins are combination molecules containing both lipids (fats) and proteins. This structure

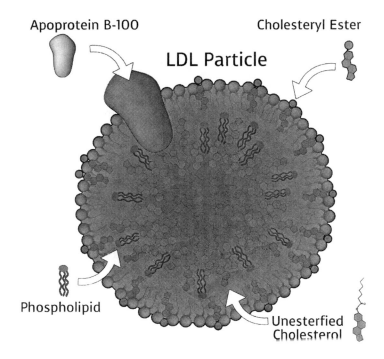

Apoprotein B-100

Cholesteryl Ester

LDL Particle

Phospholipid

Unesterfied
Cholesterol

allows fats to be transported in the bloodstream. Everyone knows oil and water do not mix; the same thing occurs in the body. Lipoproteins are like a bus that carries passengers safely inside. The passengers in this case include cholesterol, triglycerides, CoQ10, and vitamins A, D, E, and K.

There are several types of lipoproteins: LDL, HDL, VLDL, IDL, and chylomicrons. Each one of these molecules serves a life-sustaining purpose. In fact, lipoproteins were recently discovered to be an integral part of our immune system used to fight off bacterial infections.[9]

LDL stands for low-density lipoprotein. I like to think of this particle as a bus that carries cholesterol, phospholipids, and triglycerides as its passengers. The surface of the LDL contains a molecule called Apo B-100. This protein supports the structure of the LDL, helps enzymes function, and assists the LDL when parking in tissues to drop off its passengers. The LDL molecule also contains another surface protein called Apo E. This protein is also responsible for recognition of LDL around the body in areas such as the liver, endothelial cells, and just about every other cell in the body. Apo E has variants 2, 3, 4 with the 2's and 4's associated with increased cardiac risk and the 4 actually associated with increased risk of dementia. Is your doctor testing your levels of Apo B-100 and Apo E genetics?

★LIVE WELL: LDL is very important, which is the reason all animals produce it.

As mentioned above, many other nutrients are passengers on the LDL bus. The bus travels around the body to different organs where the passengers are needed. Cholesterol is needed to form cell membranes, sex hormones, cortisol, vitamin D, and the digestive bile salts. Phospholipids in the LDL are critical for cell membrane integrity and function (remember the fence). Cells talk to each other in a variety of ways and an optimally functioning cell membrane has plenty of quality phospholipids to allow for this communication. Triglycerides are passengers inside LDL and are a major source of energy for the body. The breakdown of triglycerides makes critical energy for heart and muscle function. Most doctors would never guess LDL has an antioxidant function when it responds to damaged (oxidized) vascular tissues.

BUT THE MAN ON TV SAID LDL IS BAD?

For years doctors and patients alike were taught that LDL is the "bad" cholesterol. Apparently the thinking is the human body, and most other animals, manufacture something that causes damage and disease. Isn't that insane? In reality, studies show across a wide range of LDL numbers, the risk of heart attack and stroke appear to be equal. According to the Framingham Heart study, the largest and longest running population-based study in the U.S., an LDL of 100 carries the same risk as an LDL of 160 mg/dl. Going above 160 only slightly increases risk. This is contrary to what doctors believe, but the data is very clear and has been widely available since the 1980's. A study from 2006 showed that in over 130,000 patients hospitalized with coronary artery disease, the vast majority had an LDL between 60 and 130. The highest percentile was in the group of patients with an LDL of 90.[10]

In one of the early drug trials, AFCAPS/TEXCAPS, patients with an LDL under 160 had a 5% chance of having a heart attack after 5 years follow up. Those with LDL above 160 had a 7% chance after 5 years. That is only a 2% difference. Interestingly, higher levels of LDL were not associated with a higher risk of dying, only a higher risk of heart attack.[11] This is quite different than the story we hear from doctors and advertisers who warn us that bad cholesterol kills and we need to lower it to live. As noted above, very high LDL is associated with a higher risk of heart attack, but it is only slight. We do not need drugs. There is a better way.

Everyone has a perfect LDL number appropriate for them based on their genetics. I call this the Caveman Cholesterol. What would the person's LDL level be if they lived 25,000 years ago? If a person follows the appropriate nutrition, avoids chemicals, detoxifies, and takes the correct supplements, the Caveman Cholesterol will be achieved.

★**LIVE WELL**: The goal of any person reading this book is neither a 5% or 7% chance of having a heart attack. The goal is to get near a 0% chance.

BEYOND TOTAL LDL

Hundreds of studies used the LDL-C, which is the total amount of cholesterol carried in the LDL particles. This number is a calculated number and is not typically measured directly. The fact that this number was used instead of LDL particle numbers and sizes explains why so many people form blockages with "normal" LDL-C, and why so many people with "high" LDL-C have no evidence of disease. Let me explain this critical difference further:

LDL particles travel in 2 basic types, A and B. The A is a large, fluffy LDL that floats around the body as nature intended, not causing any harm. They are doing their job delivering cholesterol and other nutrients to areas of need. In contrast, type B particles are small, dense LDL—the problem version. The small LDL started off large and fluffy, but float around the body too long. If the LDL is loaded with triglycerides (from carbs/sugar) it will continue to circulate and become smaller and prone to oxidation. This oxidation is like the rust

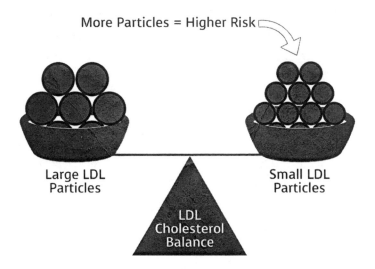

found on an old car. The oxidized, small LDL is picked up by inflammatory cells in the vessel wall, contributing to plaque formation and ultimately to coronary artery disease.

Let me further clarify this concept of large and small particles. Two people can have the same LDL-C of 100 mg/dl, but one person has 1000 large particles (which is good) and another has 2000 small particles (bad). This means their risk is totally different. People with increased amounts of small, dense LDL are at much greater risk of coronary disease. So this explains why some people with high LDL-C develop coronary artery disease and some do not. If your percentage of small, dense LDL is low, your risk is much lower than if you have a high percentage of these coronary disease-causing molecules. Know your particle numbers and sizes. This type of testing is what sets me apart from the typical cardiologist.

HDL

HDL stands for high-density lipoprotein. This lipoprotein is manufactured by the liver and is a scavenger that picks up excess cholesterol from around the body and brings it back to the liver for reprocessing. This process, called reverse cholesterol transport, actually pulls cholesterol from the inflammatory cells in the vessel wall. In an action similar to LDL, HDL delivers cholesterol to organs that create hormones and perform other cellular functions. HDL helps to inhibit: oxidation (damage) of tissues and LDL; inflammation; coagulation (blood clotting); and platelet aggregation (blood clotting). HDL inhibits damaged LDL and inflammatory cells from adhering to the endothelial membrane. All of this should serve to decrease cardiovascular risk. HDL is active in our immune system to fight off infections, and it transports lutein and zeaxanthin, naturally occurring antioxidants critical for eye health.[12]

Higher levels of HDL are associated with a decreased risk of coronary disease, and any number below 40 mg/dl in men and 50 mg/dl in women markedly increases cardiovascular risk. A person with an HDL of 25 mg/dl has four times the risk as someone with an HDL of 65,[13] all other factors equal. HDL size is also very important with the large, fluffy HDL associated with decreased risk. Some people produce a high amount of HDL, but the particles don't work. Sugar is the main culprit leading to dysfunctional HDL.

We learned from estrogen replacement studies that raising HDL does not always result in clinical benefit. Niacin raises HDL, but the pharmaceuticals that specifically increase HDL were a miserable failure. Good nutrition, exercise, and chemical avoidance will raise HDL and improve their ability to remove cholesterol from coronary plaque. Alcohol can raise HDL, but I do not recommend its use. HDL2b is the form that has scavenged the most cholesterol from around the body, including the plaque. HDL2b is tested by advanced laboratories and higher levels are an indication reverse transport is functioning well.

TRIGLYCERIDES

Triglycerides (TRG's) are molecules of fat, which are found in food and also produced by the liver. When we take a bite out of salmon, the fat is in the triglyceride form. Three carbon atoms make up the glycerol backbone with 3 fatty acid groups attached. These fatty acid groups are monounsaturated, polyunsaturated, and saturated fats. TRG's are broken down in the intestines and easily absorbed. The liver packages triglycerides to use for energy or store as fat. TRG's travel inside lipoproteins, such as LDL and HDL. The more carbohydrates, sugar, and excess calories consumed, the more triglycerides are stored as fat.

Elevated blood levels of triglycerides are associated with an increased risk of coronary disease. A meta-analysis from 2007, including over 200,000 patients, concluded triglycerides are an independent risk factor for coronary artery disease (CAD).[14] As the lipoprotein particles LDL and HDL travel around the body, triglyceride passengers are removed and the particles get smaller and become damaged. The small, damaged LDL particles are the ones easily incorporated into the blood vessel wall and into a coronary plaque. Therefore, the higher the triglycerides, the more CAD. Omega-3 fish oil and niacin are beneficial in lowering triglycerides levels, but going after the cause should always be the first move. The causes here are carbohydrates and sugar. Most labs use the fasting value of 150 mg/dl as normal, but I prefer my patients get under 100 mg/dl.

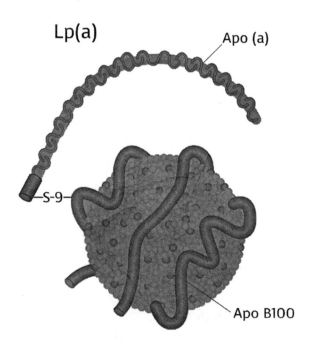

DO YOU KNOW ABOUT LP(A)?

Lp(a) is similar to LDL, but is a nasty little bugger that causes a lot of damage. You can blame your parents for this one because it is genetically linked. Lp(a) consists of the apo B-100 protein I mentioned before, attached to apo(a) protein. Young patients with heart disease usually have elevated Lp(a) levels, which is likely a major factor in their early onset and aggressive blockages.

Lp(a) looks like plasminogen, a protein involved in clot prevention. Years ago in the emergency room, we used a clot buster called TPA when a heart attack victim arrived. TPA stands for tissue plasminogen activator. Since the Lp(a) structure is similar to plasminogen, it diminishes the conversion of plasminogen to its active enzyme form, plasmin. Plasmin is like a tiny "Pacman" gobbling up clots, so with decreased levels of plasmin your blood clot risk is increased. The problems don't stop there. The Lp(a) particle easily oxidizes (damaged), crosses the endothelium (lining) of the blood vessel, and increases inflammation, which ultimately leads to blockage and plaque rupture. Lp(a) also appears to interfere with blood vessel dilation. Lp(a) is no laughing matter.[15]

Mechanisms of Lp(a) damage:

- Avidly taken up by inflammatory cells in plaque
- Leads to inflammatory cell recruitment to plaque
- Interferes with plasminogen; therefore, interferes with clot breakdown
- Impairs vasodilation
- Promotes smooth muscle cell proliferation in plaque
- Impairs barrier function of endothelial cells

Lp(a) levels are difficult to lower, but one proven way is by eating saturated fat. Yes, animal fats and coconut oil drop Lp(a) by 10% on average.16 Don't look to Lipitor for help because trials using statin therapy do not show any consistent benefit in lowering Lp(a) levels. Hormone replacement therapy in women has proven effective, but I would not recommend its use specifically to lower Lp(a). The go-to supplement in this situation is time-release niacin, which reduces levels by 20-30%. There is promising data on N-acetyl cysteine, vitamin C, and L-carnitine. Because of the increased clotting risk associated with Lp(a), it is my personal recommendation to use nattokinase or lumbrokinase along with other natural blood thinners such as omega-3 fish oil, garlic, and vitamins C and E.

★LIVE WELL: Supplements are beneficial, but the most important thing is a healthy Paleo diet.

CASE STUDY

Jim P. is a 37-year old guy who came to me because he was told his cholesterol was high. His doctor wanted to put him on pharmaceuticals, but he was not comfortable with that recommendation. Jim's total cholesterol was 243 with an LDL of 167. The knee-jerk, drug company response is to prescribe statins. However, I looked more in depth at his blood with advanced lipid analysis and found his LDL particle count was in a decent range, his protective HDL particles were high, and his triglycerides were 140. He had normal levels of Lp(a). We talked about Paleo nutrition and I had Jim start off with a one-week juice cleanse. Three months later we repeated Jim's blood tests, which revealed even lower LDL particles but with a larger size. His total LDL actually dropped to 133, which is likely his "Caveman Cholesterol." What I call Caveman Cholesterol is really the cholesterol number for someone who was walking around the planet 50,000 years ago. Jim no longer sees his original cardiologist.

ACTION PLAN

1. LDL carries cholesterol, vitamins, Co Q 10, and other nutrients around the body.
2. HDL is very beneficial, but it can be damaged easily from sugar and toxins.
3. Know your particle numbers and sizes.
4. Lp(a) is a nasty player.
5. LDL does not cause disease. Whatever is leading to small, damaged LDL is the real cause.

As this chapter has shown, it is very clear cholesterol, LDL, HDL, and triglycerides all serve a purpose. We evolved over millions of years and contain these molecules for a reason. Without them, animal life does not exist. Yet the medical establishment continues to treat lipids as the enemy. The quest to discover more drugs to combat cholesterol seems never-ending. We need to realize cholesterol does not cause disease. What does cause disease is eating unhealthy foods like sugar, wheat, soy, and corn. Living in a world filled with air pollutants, heavy metals, toxic laundry products, and plastics also leads to health problems. What we call disease is really the body's response to these poisons. Your typical M.D. does not understand this, which is why it is of extreme importance to find a health care provider who does.

If we've been misled about cholesterol, what else is untrue? Now, let's learn the TRUTH about nutrition and how to avoid the chemicals and toxins that CAUSE disease.

⤜——▷ Chapter 3 ◁——⤛

LET'S EAT PALEO

"Let Food Be Thy Medicine."
—Hippocrates

Every society in the history of the world ate meat and/or seafood. Thousands of years ago, during the Paleolithic Age, humans were hunter-gathers, eating the foods available to pick or kill. These foods allowed man to thrive without all the chronic diseases we see today. Some researchers propose meat, seafood, and fat consumption led to bigger brains, capable of complex thought, communication, and other advanced behaviors. Thousands of research papers have documented the Paleo diet. We do know grain intake was minimal, animals were not milked, and sugar was non-existent, aside from a rare honey treat or seasonal fruit. Paleo nutrition involves a modern approach to the hunter-gatherer diet.

Around the world, Paleo cultures ate a variety of foods. This is well documented by explorers and scientists. The food available to our ancestors depended on

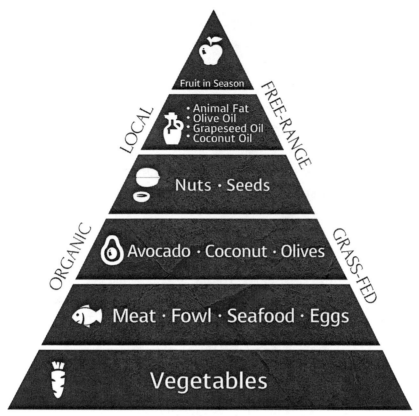

THE DRS. WOLFSON PALEO PYRAMID

their location. Obviously, one spot on the globe grew plenty of avocados while another location produced more nuts and seeds. But the foundation of Paleo nutrition was the same: vegetables, meat, seafood, nuts, seeds, eggs, and fruit. There was no portion control. Our ancestors did not catch a wild salmon and try to determine a four-ounce portion. Remember, Paleo is not a diet, but a way of eating which coincided with our evolution. It is what we are designed to eat. Diets are fads such as vegan, South Beach, and Engine #2.

NO MORE EXCUSES

When it comes to Paleo, many people are turned off by the name and recent media hype. Some think they cannot follow the plan, and therefore tune out.

But my job is to tell people the best way to eat. How much you follow my advice is up to you. 100% adherence will lead to 100% results. Some people may still consume organic dairy, gluten-free grain, and organic sugars. But if you want to enjoy the best health, keep these cheat foods to a minimum. If you suffer from heart disease, cancer, or autoimmune conditions, please stay 100% gluten free. All cheat foods MUST be organic.

> ★LIVE WELL: Paleo nutrition is based upon vegetables, meat, seafood, nuts, seeds, eggs, and a small amount of fruit—no grain, dairy, or sugar.

PALEO PROOF

Before we discuss the Paleo foods, I want to offer some evidence proving its benefits. There are several comparison studies between Paleo nutrition and other diets. Lindeberg and associates reported a study in 2007 in which a group of 29 patients with heart disease and type 2 diabetes were placed on either a Paleolithic diet or a Mediterranean diet. While both diets worked, the weight loss after 12 weeks was significantly greater in the Paleolithic diet group.[17]

The above study, demonstrating Paleo trumped the Mediterranean diet, is very compelling. Given the fact the Mediterranean diet was superior to a low fat diet in the landmark PREDIMED trial, imagine what Paleo could do.[18] In PREDIMED, over 7000 patients were divided into two groups. One group was advised to eat a low-fat diet based on the recommendations of the American Heart Association. The other group was taught to consume a diet with fish, poultry, vegetables, nuts, seeds, and olive oil. The results were very impressive in favor of the Mediterranean group as total heart attacks and strokes were reduced by 30%!

A 2009 study compared the Paleo diet to a diabetic diet (low in fat with increased whole grain intake). The Paleo group was advised to avoid all dairy products, all grain products including rice and corn, all legumes including peanuts, and all sugar except fruit. The results were impressively in favor of Paleo for improving blood sugar, triglycerides, and raising HDL. Blood pressure, weight loss, and waist circumference were better in the Paleo group.[19]

In 1984, ten full-blooded Australian Aborigines with diabetes agreed to be tested before and after living for seven weeks as hunter-gatherers. Previously, these ten overweight, middle-aged people had been living in modern cities and ate a standard diet. With a diet two-thirds animal-based, the group averaged 18 pounds of weight loss and markedly improved their blood sugar and fasting insulin levels. Triglycerides were reduced by 75%!

★**LIVE WELL**: Paleo beats Mediterranean and all other diets.

Pretty simple, isn't it? Go back to the basics and you will discover the cure for diabetes. It is sad that some people prefer pills and insulin injections to normalize their blood sugar, never understanding that pills and injections do little to lower cardiovascular risk.[20] Now let's sink our teeth into the foods our ancestors have enjoyed for millions of years.

PALEO FOODS

Vegetables

The foundation of a healthy nutrition plan and my Paleo Pyramid is vegetables. Except for the Chocolate Chip Cookie Diet, every book on nutrition stresses the importance of eating plants. The only thing the government Food Plate gets right is recommending many servings of veggies per day. By harnessing the power of the sun in packets called chlorophyll, plants are packed with nutrition. I start my day with a greens drink, either freshly juiced or reconstituted powder. Lunch is usually a large salad containing a variety of greens, nuts, seeds, and olives topped with olive oil, lemon juice, and sea salt. Dinner is more salad, cooked veggies, and meat or seafood. Organic vegetables are present at every meal. If organic vegetables are not in season or available for a particular meal, don't eat the pesticide version. Many restaurants claim to serve organic when available. Get a clue chef: if organic spinach is not available, don't serve spinach!

★**LIVE WELL**: Start your day off with a greens drink. If you are still hungry, eat bacon, eggs, avocado, nuts, and seeds. Create your own "cereal" with nuts, seeds, coconut, raw cacao, and homemade nut milk.

So what makes our little green friends critical to good health? First, vegetables are loaded with fiber, a great vehicle for keeping our bowels moving. Attention! Stagnant bowels allow the food to rot in your colon, with inflammation and cancer sure to follow. Second, the fiber in the vegetables serves as a prebiotic, fostering the growth and health of the good bacteria that colonize the colon. When you house a healthy number of these guys, you are going to live a long life. I cannot stress the importance of gastrointestinal health enough, because most disease starts in the gut. Third, vegetables are packed with vitamins and minerals (including calcium), phytonutrients, and antioxidants.

★LIVE WELL: Use a greens powder daily or make a fresh juice from celery, cucumber, cabbage, kale, cilantro, parsley, carrots, beets, etc.

Go for a variety of greens such as spinach, dandelion, kale, chard, and collards. All of these can be diced up and put into a salad. There are many different types of lettuce and other greens such as arugula that add tremendous flavor. Another favorite of mine is sorrel, which tastes like lemon. Broccoli, cabbage, celery, cucumber, fennel, cauliflower, parsley, cilantro, carrots, and beets add to a variety of tastes and textures. Making your own sprouts is a fun hobby with extraordinary health benefits. Broccoli sprouts are major cancer fighters (check out sproutpeople.org). I add a tablespoon of spirulina and chlorella, two forms of blue-green algae, to my salad. Both of these amazing "superfoods" are loaded with protein and chlorophyll, the powerhouse that converts sunshine into food energy (read more on these two in Chapter 16). Most of the above foods can be steamed, sautéed, or used in baked dishes. Cooking destroys some nutrients, yet accentuates others, which is why it's a good idea to eat both ways. Two-thirds raw is a good rule of thumb.

Root veggies, such as carrots, turmeric, radishes, turnips, onions, garlic, and ginger, are excellent. In Paleo times, potatoes were found and consumed, but when cooked they become sugar bombs. If you are trying to lose weight or have elevated blood sugar, cooked potatoes are not your friends. You can eat sweet potatoes and yams raw. These yield excellent fiber and are also considered a prebiotic, as healthy bacteria thrive on these tubers.

★LIVE WELL: As you eat or drink, visualize the food cleansing, nourishing, and healing your body.

There is a class of vegetables deserving special mention called nightshades, named because they grow best at night. Tomatoes, peppers, eggplant, zucchini, and squash are in this category. Unfortunately, many people unknowingly react to these vegetables and manifest symptoms from skin disorders, such as eczema, to arthritic conditions. When you are following Paleo but still not feeling at your best, nightshades could be the enemy. In general, I limit this category of food.

Meat

Few topics stir up controversy quite like eating meat. Despite the fact humans have been omnivores for millions of years, many health "authorities" want to vilify our ancestral food. Whenever a study attacks meat consumption, you need to look at the source. Studies concluding veganism is preferable do not account for the fact that vegans are a health conscious group (just wrong about meat and seafood). Vegans tend to avoid smoking, consistently exercise, consume vitamins, and are more chemical-conscious compared to the population who eat fast food and drink soda pop. A study from 1996 found health conscious people enjoy a 50% lower risk of heart disease, whether they eat meat or not.[21] Researchers believe the human brain achieved its greatness only after we started eating meat and seafood. When meat is from a free-range, healthy and happy animal, enjoying its native foods, the consumer gains extraordinary health benefits.

★LIVE WELL: Women who eat meat build more muscle than vegetarians.

Some things are only found in meat

Nutrients from animal sources

1. B12 is critical for brain function, energy, and detoxification. You cannot get B12 from plants.
2. Carnosine functions as a powerful anti-oxidant, enhances athletic performance, and provides protection against many diseases. Prevents glycation damage from sugar and is 50% lower in vegetarians.[22]
3. Creatine forms an energy reserve in the muscles and brain and is found only in animal foods. Low creatine leads to reduced physical and mental performance.
4. Meat and seafood contain beneficial fats such as EPA/DHA and many more. Plants do not contains these fats.
5. Vegans are often deficient in zinc, iron, and riboflavin (B2).
6. Vegans are low in vitamin D3. While sunshine makes vitamin D, many areas have insufficient UVB sunrays for most of the year. Only D3 from animal sources will significantly raise D3.
7. Vegans get beta-carotene from plants, but the body must convert this to vitamin A. In many people, this conversion is inadequate. Only animal foods contain available vitamin A.
8. Vegans are low in taurine, an essential nutrient for heart health.[23]

★ **LIVE WELL**: *Meat eaters produce more testosterone compared to vegetarians.*[24]

When discussing meat, I am referring to cow, bison, elk, pig, lamb, turkey, chicken, and wild game that are free range and grass-fed. A healthy animal consumes its native diet. This means humanely raised, grass-fed animals. I am not saying, "Go to Burger King and eat a double Whopper, hold the bun." Cows and other mammals eat grass. Turkeys and chickens eat grass, forage for seeds, and eat bugs. All animals should be in a stress-free environment, basking in sunshine and fresh air. Their living conditions should be similar to what they would experience in the wild. Read one of my favorites,

Upton Sinclair's *The Jungle*, to understand where animal cruelty in the food industry started.

★**LIVE WELL**: Meat eaters are at lower risk of an osteoporotic fracture.[25]

There is plenty of proof a grass-fed animal is more healthy, not that we need any proof, since it makes perfect sense. Nonetheless, an article published in 2006 compared grass-fed to grain-fed cattle. The grass-fed animals had higher levels of beneficial omega-3 fats and conjugated linoleic acid.[26] Several studies suggest cows eating grass-based diets contain elevated precursors for vitamins A and E, as well as cancer-fighting antioxidants such as glutathione and superoxide dismutase activity, compared to grain-fed cows.[27]

Several factors go into raising sickly animals, including antibiotic abuse, synthetic hormones, stressful living situations, and unhealthy feeding practices. Antibiotics were created to treat life-threatening infections. Nowadays, they are added to animal feed, as a way to prevent infections. The Food and Drug Administration continues to allow dozens of antibiotics to be used in livestock feed. This is despite findings from the National Defense Resources Council that the drugs could expose humans to deadly, antibiotic-resistant bacteria. Cows get sick when they are fed grain (so do humans). They get fat and are more likely to injure themselves (so do humans). They are essentially malnourished, causing their immune systems to not function well (so are humans). Factory farm animals do not get sunshine and are under constant stress.

★**LIVE WELL**: Do not eat tortured animal products at restaurants, a friend's house, sporting event, etc.

Growth hormones are injected into animals to make them grow quicker and larger. The faster an animal grows, the sooner you can sell it. The bigger the animal, the more there is to sell. According to a European Union scientific committee, the use of growth hormones in beef production poses a potential risk to human health.[28] The committee questioned whether hormone residues in the meat of growth-enhanced animals can disrupt human hormone balance, causing developmental problems, interfering with the reproductive system, and even leading to the development of breast, prostate and colon cancers. The hormones certainly wind up in dairy products, which children consume. It is no surprise when an eight-year-old girl enters puberty or a young boy has a real mustache from milk. Our friends at Monsanto created the genetically engineered growth hormone and use it based on scant testing performed on rats. The health ramifications may never be fully recognized.

★**LIVE WELL**: Buy grass-fed meat at your local butcher or farmers market.

Yuck...not liver!

The internal organs are actually the most prized part of the animal. Our ancestors ate the liver, kidneys, spleen, and thyroid first, not the filet or rib eye. Carnivores such as sharks, lions, etc. will go after the liver of its prey, then eat the other internal organs. The innards are loaded with vitamins, minerals, protein, and healthy fats. Bone marrow is a delicacy of delicious heart-healthy fat. Boiled bones make a healing broth packed with minerals including calcium. Liver, kidney, and other organ meats can be blended and added to ground meat, or served as an excellent addition to soup. Ironically, these portions are the healthiest, yet the cheapest cuts. We add liver to our homemade chicken soup recipe.

★**LIVE WELL**: You will get plenty of calcium from Paleo sources.

What about processed meat?

There is much debate about the health ramifications of processed meats such as bacon, sausage, and hot dogs. Of course, any meat from a tortured animal, fed grain and loaded with hormones and antibiotics, is considered toxic and not on the nutrition plan. But I think processed meats are fine in moderation, meaning one to two times per week. Just read the ingredients and watch for additives like sugar or soy, and avoid smoked meats if possible. Ask your local grocer or butcher about grass-fed options. They more we demand, the more companies will produce.

Another debate surrounds the nitrates and nitrites added to meat as preservatives. Claims are made that they cause cancer and neurologic disorders such as Parkinson's. Fortunately, based on recent studies, those claims have been proven false.[29] The reality is that the human body naturally produces nitrates and nitrites, infinitely more than what are found in food. Speaking of nitrates, vegetables, such as beets and arugula, are loaded with nitrates that cause vasodilation (increased blood vessel size) and lower blood pressure. Processed meats claiming nitrate-free status are misleading and contain the same amount of nitrates, just from a natural source, such as beet or celery juice. Bacon, sausage, and hot dogs can be an excellent source of quick nutrition, as long as they are from grass-fed and free-range animals.

★LIVE WELL: How much meat you eat is up to you, but everyone should eat some meat and seafood.

Seafood

Seafood and the omega-3 fats it contains are well documented to promote tremendous cardiovascular benefits. A review in 2006 found those individuals eating fish one to two times per week had a 36% lower risk of coronary artery disease.[30] Those people with the highest omega-3 levels enjoy the best cardiovascular outcomes.[31] Fish consumption is associated with a decreased risk of carotid artery blockage, the main vessel that sends blood to your brain.[32] The more disease in the carotid, the higher the risk of stroke. Fish intake is associated with a 20% lower risk of diabetes.[33] Vegans have very low levels of omega-3 in their cells.[34]

Seafood in the diet is a tough proposition because the waters are polluted, so choices are limited. The only seafood I recommend is wild salmon and small fish, such as anchovy, sardines, smelts, and herring. Tuna, shark, swordfish, and other big fish are out since they are loaded with mercury and other toxins. Wild fish, such as sea bass, perch, trout, and Mahi Mahi, should be consumed sparingly. The same goes for shellfish. If you know the lake or river is clean, feel free to eat the fish. Never eat farm-raised seafood. Google the images of these farms and you will be mortified to see beautiful creatures swimming in their own filth while consuming unnatural food and antibiotics.

Anchovies taste great and our kids love them. If you or your loved one is not so keen on the taste, hide it in salad dressing after blending with olive oil and lemon. Buy anchovies in glass bottles to avoid the BPA and plastic from cans (more on BPA and plastic in Chapter 8). Sardines are found whole and fresh occasionally, but we usually have to eat them from a can. Find BPA-free cans, and even then, consume sparingly due to the plastic liner and metal.

★LIVE WELL: To counteract the heavy metals found in seafood, I recommend the blue-green algae, chlorella, to bind the toxins. Drink after your meal and the metals will be safely carried out the other end.

Nuts and Seeds

Nuts and seeds are a large part of the Mediterranean diet and one of the main sources of the diet's success. They are loaded with vitamins, minerals, and healthy fats. In fact, most nuts are about 50% fat by volume. Generous amounts of vitamin E are found in most nuts. They are a significant source of calcium, another reason we do not need dairy for this nutrient. Nuts contain abundant protein from 18 different amino acids. Nuts and seeds provide fiber, so we do not need wheat or other grains to move our bowels. Different nuts contain different nutrients, so variety is key here.

In a study published in 2011, nut consumption was associated with decreased weight, waist circumference, blood pressure, higher HDL, and lower blood sugar. Despite the fact nuts are high in calories, those who consumed the most had the lowest rates of obesity.[35] The only way to gain weight is by eating carbs and sugar. Additional studies demonstrate nuts and seeds lower oxidative stress, inflammation, and improve vascular reactivity. Cancer risk also appears to be lower in those with the most nut/seed consumption.[36] In 2013, the NEJM reported those who ate the most nuts lived the longest.[37]

Some of the benefit regarding nuts and seeds may be in the way the gut microbiome is affected. Bacteria in our intestines is critical to overall health, and a recent study confirmed that almonds and pistachios increase the amount of beneficial flora.[38] Fortunately, nuts and seeds do not cause the colon condition, diverticulitis. In fact, a study in 2008 from *JAMA* revealed those who eat the most amounts of nuts and seeds report the least amount of diverticulitis.[39] Diverticulitis (pockets of infection in the colon) is from non-Paleo foods such as grain, dairy, and sugar. Tell that to your doctor.

★**LIVE WELL**: Peanuts are a bean and not on the Paleo nutrition plan. They are highly allergenic, inhibit digestion, and contain a mold that produces aflatoxin, which can lead to liver damage and even cirrhosis.

Just about any nut or seed makes for an excellent snack. I often eat a mixture of raw nuts for breakfast with added coconut flakes and homemade nut milk. Add nuts and seeds to salad for a protein and fat boost that fills you up. It is doubtful nuts and seeds were historically consumed in mass quantity. Imagine yourself in Paleo days encountering a walnut tree. You would find the shell and have to crack it, which is no easy task. Then you need to pick the nut from the shell, which again is not easy and fraught with injury risk. This whole process is time consuming and labor intensive, certainly when compared to sitting on the couch with a bag of mixed nuts eating them as fast as your hand will move. The shell seems to be nature's way of preventing us from eating too much, too fast.

Don't run out and eat a bag of almonds just yet. Nuts and seeds produce enzyme inhibitors that can interfere with digestion and inhibit mineral absorption. To combat these troublesome molecules, it is recommended to soak RAW nuts in water for a few hours. This simulates rain on a fallen nut and allows it to germinate, minimizing the anti-nutrients. The larger the nut or seed, the longer you need to soak it. Discard the water afterwards. At the risk of being accused of repetition, nuts and seeds must be organic. Pesticides kill bugs and they kill us.

★**LIVE WELL**: Raw nuts and seeds lower your risk of heart disease, cancer, and diverticulitis.

Eggs

For many years, the egg has been vilified as the prototypical dangerous food that causes coronary disease and heart attacks. Health authorities told us the cholesterol in eggs, along with saturated fat, was something to avoid. The Food Pyramid (or sick pyramid as I call it) had us limit this horrible orb. The TRUTH is, an egg is a cocoon for a baby chicken, which cannot grow to life without the cholesterol and dozens of vitamins and minerals it contains. The saturated fats in eggs are necessary for the cellular growth of the chicken, much like the saturated fat in breast milk is necessary for human growth. Mother Nature wouldn't try to hurt us, would she? Every animal goes after another animal's eggs; sounds like they are on to something.

There are many studies refuting a link between cholesterol in foods and heart disease. Shockingly, after 40 years of the government and doctors telling patients not to eat cholesterol food, an abrupt change in recommendations appears to be on the horizon. The 2015 guidelines, set for release by the federal government, will likely reflect that saturated fat and cholesterol should be part of a healthy diet. Stay tuned.

Eggs raise HDL.40 The more eggs you eat, the lower your risk of diabetes.41 The egg yolk is a wonderful source of vitamins A (critical for eye health), D (strengthens bones, prevents heart and neurological disease, normalizes blood pressure), and E (antioxidant and cancer fighter). Eggs are high in protein and contain zero carbs or sugars. Eggs are high in several B vitamins, iron, selenium, and other minerals. Eggs are like a natural multivitamin.

★**LIVE WELL**: Eggs do not contribute to heart attacks.

All eggs are not created equal. When I recommend eggs, I am referring to those from free range chickens that get plenty of sunshine, are allowed to forage, and eat bugs. Eggs should come from chickens that are not stuffed with soy, corn, or other grains, as these birds are not healthy. The best scenario is to raise chickens like we do. Birds are omnivores, eating meat, seafood, bugs, nuts, seeds, and veggies. If we need more eggs, we buy from a farmer who raises free range chickens that eat bugs, seeds, and veggies. My favorite store brand is Vital Farms, but do your own research.

Don't ask the typical doctor who has ZERO training in nutrition, or listen to a talking head on TV. Go with your gut and the fact that humans ate eggs for millions of years. Remember, eat the whole egg—consuming just the whites will rob your body of B vitamins. Lastly, cook your eggs on a low temperature, leaving the yolk soft. Cooking food at high temperatures will turn a healthy fat bad! So ditch your oatmeal and skip the Cheerios. For a healthy and satisfying start to your day, eat some eggs. I do.

Avocado

One of my favorite foods, and a staple of a healthy diet, is the avocado. This delicious orb is actually a fruit, not a vegetable. It is packed full of nutrients, fat, and fiber. The avocado is easy to travel with. When I was working weekends and refused to eat the poison in the hospital cafeteria, I would pack an avocado and a can of sardines as my lunch. Stories on hospital food could fill another book. Seriously, hospitals serve pancakes with sugar-free syrup to diabetes patients. Again, a hospital is one of the most disgusting and toxic places on the planet. Sadly, most women give birth there, instead of at home.

Back to the beauty and many varieties of avocado. The Hass is the most common, though the Reed has been popping up more recently. The Reed is much larger than the Hass and has a creamy taste. An avocado is easy to "hide" in recipes such as puddings. Add a little raw cacao and honey and the kids will never know what they just ate. Avocado is an excellent first food for babies, as they do not require any teeth to chew.

Avocado is actually mostly water by volume. The second biggest component is fat. The monounsaturated fat known as oleic acid constitutes the majority; it lowers LDL, raises HDL, and decreases blood pressure. In fact, one study reported a 22% reduction in LDL and 11% increase in HDL with avocado consumption.[42] This may be from the high content of beta-sitosterols. Another study demonstrated avocado consumption decreases oxidized LDL (the nasty kind) while increasing non-oxidized levels. This is likely due to the fact that avocado is high in vitamins C and E, nutrients proven to slow atherosclerosis. The fat in the avocado helps with absorption of vitamins A, D, E, and K. There is also evidence this food prevents cancer.[43]

> ★LIVE WELL: Eat 3-4 avocados per week. They reduce damaged LDL particles.

When you tell patients to avoid grain, one of the first things they worry about is how they will move their bowels. Well, the avocado is loaded with 5-10 grams of fiber depending on the size. In addition, it is high in magnesium and is a much better source of potassium than a banana, which is high in sugar. The sugar content of an avocado is very close to zero and has no impact on blood sugar. Of course, antioxidants and phytochemicals are present in this food, which also decrease cardiovascular risk and are natural anti-inflammatories. Finally, the B vitamins in the avocado help to lower homocysteine, a molecule associated with heart disease, cancer, and dementia.

> ★LIVE WELL: Any diet change can lead to constipation. Eat Paleo and drink plenty of water. Your bowels will start to move.

Coconut

The coconut is an amazing food falsely vilified over the years because of its high saturated fat content. Islands in the South Pacific consume 50% of their calories from this food, yet rarely suffer from heart disease. In the 1970's the corn and soy industries promoted misinformation regarding the coconut. These two industries had the most to gain from the demise of the coconut, especially coconut oil. The fact that the coconut and its oil are higher in saturated fat is actually a benefit, making the coconut more stable in cooking, since saturated fat limits oxidation damage and prolongs shelf life. Please read *The Coconut Diet* by Cherie Calbom for an in-depth review of the history of coconuts, the smear campaign, and the real story behind the benefits.

Coconuts are high in fiber. Coconut oil is mostly lauric acid and caprylic acid. Lauric acid is a large constituent of human breast milk, which by definition makes it healthy. Lauric acid prevents cancer,[44] raises HDL,[45] and fights bacterial infections.[46] Caprylic acid also confers similar benefits. Recently, coconut oil was found to have a beneficial effect on the lipid profile of pre-menopausal women in the Philippines. HDL levels were higher among coconut oil users.[47]

★**LIVE WELL**: Coconuts are a great source of saturated fat, fiber, and acids that fight cancer, raise HDL, and fight infections.

You can eat the coconut meat by itself, blend it into a "yogurt," or ferment as kefir. Coconut flakes are a great snack; our kids love them, and they can be added to your nut "cereal." Coconut oil is great for slow cooking your eggs, baking, and applying on your skin. I use it for aftershave. If you drink coconut water, do so in moderation. It is high in sugar, a fact that, along with its high level of electrolytes, made it a useful intravenous fluid. Coconut milk and other canned products should be avoided for the same reasons all canned products should be avoided—contamination from plastic and the leeching of metal.

Fruit

In Paleo days, fruits were wild berries and Crab apples only available in the late summer/early fall when ripe. Today, many people drink a fruit smoothie for breakfast, eat fruit after meals, and fruit every night at bedtime. That is an awful lot of sugar. Fruit is shipped from all over the world, so any time of the year you can enjoy cherries from Chile or pineapples from Hawaii. This is obviously unnatural and not very Paleo. Transportation of fruit across state lines usually involves pesticides even when organic, let alone when the produce comes from out of the country. The word fumigated comes to mind in this context.

Sure, there are beneficial antioxidants in fruit, but the risk associated with the excessive sugar intake likely outweighs any benefits. Vegetables, herbs, and spices contain enough antioxidants to counteract the toxins we are exposed to on a daily basis. If we need extra antioxidant support based on blood analysis, supplements can be added. The sugar in the fruit perpetuates the addiction, so you are looking for more sugar all day long. One piece/serving of fruit per day maximum is my mantra. A cleanse is a great way to heal your body and should be done without sugar—therefore no fruit. If you are trying to lose weight, get rid of the fruit. Avocado, coconut, and olives are examples of fruits you can eat liberally. They are high in fat and low in sugar, which is a tremendous combination for health.

> ★LIVE WELL: Fruit is usually loaded with pesticides and is high in sugar; stick with vegetables for weight-loss and better overall nutrition.

Fermented foods

Probiotics are recommended for everyone at every age. Literally meaning "pro-life," probiotics are the beneficial bacteria that colonize our gastrointestinal tract. In fact, the number of bacteria in our gut outnumbers the number of cells in our body by 10:1. Most of our immune system actually resides in our intestines. 21st century health is all about GI health. If the gut is in good shape, you will avoid much disease.

When probiotic supplements are recommended, we usually talk about billions of bacteria. Unfortunately, even the best products may not contain the stated number on the bottle because the bacteria die. Now, we still recommend probiotic supplements daily, but nothing is as important as cultured vegetables. One serving of this food contains trillions of bacteria. For thousands of years, the human diet contained fermented foods such as kimchi, sauerkraut, and even fermented dairy. The Japanese consume fermented soy in the form of natto.

There are a few excellent companies selling fermented veggies such as Rejuvenative Foods and Firefly. They go very well topped on burgers and hotdogs or on their own. Another option is to make your own. It is kind of like a high school lab experiment that is very rewarding. For further reading on fermented foods, please read *Wild Fermentation* by Sandor Katz.

Herbs and Spices

The list here is long and there are many excellent books written on this subject. Bottom line is we need to get herbs and spices into our diet as much as possible. They contain tremendous antioxidants and nutrients that protect against heart disease, cancer, and brain disorders. Many spices are antimicrobial and fight bacteria, viruses, candida and other yeasts, as well as parasites. In fact, many effective nutritional supplements that fight intestinal infections use high doses of herbs to kill off unwanted inhabitants. Some of my favorites include thyme, sage, turmeric, oregano, basil, and rosemary. Every time I eat eggs or meat, I add herbs and spices to the recipe. They add flavor, but most importantly, they counteract any negative effects from cooking. Just go to your local grocer and check out the spice section. Buy a wide variety, which are labeled organic, and create your own recipes. You cannot mess this up, so get creative.

One spice gaining a lot of notoriety is turmeric, a root vegetable that is the base for curry powder. The literature and studies regarding curcumin, a compound found in turmeric, are very compelling. I use this supplement with most of the patients in my practice and see amazing results. A recent study showed curcumin reduced a slew of cardiovascular risk factors in patients with diabetes.[48] Another recent study demonstrated curcumin lowers inflammation as measured by hs-CRP.[49] Elevations of this blood marker are highly correlated with cardiac risk. Supplements are great and my Top 20 are discussed in Chapter 16, so definitely add turmeric to your cooking regimen. For the best absorption, make sure turmeric is added to meals that contain fat.[50]

★**LIVE WELL**: Herbs and spices contain antioxidants and nutrients that fight bacteria and protect against heart disease, cancer, and brain disorders.

Oils and Fats

Fats and oils are actually the same thing. When the temperature is warm enough, fat liquefies into oil. Cool it back down, and the solid fat returns. When it comes to frying eggs, I use coconut oil or animal fats, such as beef tallow, pork lard, or duck fat. I save bacon grease in a container to use at another time to cook eggs. For an occasional treat, we make sweet potato fries using duck fat. Adding spices such as paprika and cayenne give the sweets a major kick, while adding critically important antioxidants.

We top our salads with olive or grape seed oil. Olive oil should be extra virgin, organic, and cold, first pressed. Olive oil makes up a large part of the highly protective Mediterranean diet. The data on the health benefits of olive oil are monumental. Only the crazy, fat-restrictive diets limit consumption of this proven health food.

Oil is pure fat, but you will lose fat and weight eating it. Other oils such as avocado and almond are beneficial, but are rarely found in glass bottles. Once again, we only consume products out of glass, never metal or plastic. Of course, hydrogenated oils are poison and we NEVER consume soybean, canola, or corn oils because they are usually GMO and definitely not Paleo. Again, read Kayla Daniel's *The Whole Soy Story*.

CASE STUDY

When Marion P. came to see me, he was well over 500 pounds. His plan was to go for gastric bypass surgery and he needed a cardiologist to okay him for the procedure. I finished my history and exam on Marion and gave him my approval for the gastric bypass. On parting, I jotted down a list of Paleo approved foods, along with my suggestion that he follow the diet and skip the surgery. I never saw Marion again.

Then one day, three years later, I received a letter in the mail. It contained a before and after picture of Marion along with a copy of my Paleo nutrition directions. He never had the gastric bypass surgery and lost over 300 pounds on his own!

ACTION PLAN

Paleo nutrition is what our ancestors ate for millions of years. Any other diet is an experiment. Don't be a guinea pig. Go with what worked for humans in the past, and led us to be the conscious beings we are today. My thousands of patients are a testimonial that Paleo works in a modern society. My patients feel great and their blood tests demonstrate a marked improvement. Check out our website, The DrsWolfson.com, for some delicious recipes.

Paleo Foods:

1. Vegetables
2. Grass fed meats, free range poultry and wild game
3. Wild seafood such as salmon, anchovy, herring, and sardines. Shellfish once per month.
4. Eggs, avocado, coconut
5. Nuts and seeds
6. Herbs and spices
7. Animal fats and coconut oil for cooking
8. Olive oil, nut oils, avocado oil, and grapeseed oil if unheated
9. Fermented foods
10. Occasional, seasonal fruit

ɲUTRITION:
WHERE DID WE ɠO WɌONG?

"You can say I'm a dreamer, well I'm not the only one."
—John Lennon

E volution is the process of change from a simple form to something more complex. Scientists believe that over millions of years, we evolved from small bacteria floating in the sea. Modern human evolution is often considered the period of time over the last 3-4 million years. During that time, we changed from an ape-like mammal to our current species. We used fire and tools for over a million years. Evidence of social structure and civilization is over 50,000 years old. Ten thousand years ago, the Agricultural Revolution began and the world was transformed from 100% hunter-gatherers to farm-based, agricultural communities. Sadly, the last 100 years has seen the industrialization of our food supply led by processing, pesticides, and the addition of mass quantities of sugar and artificial ingredients. Most recently, we are faced with another enemy—genetically modified foods.

Imagine the lifestyle of our ancestors from 25,000 years ago. This would represent about 1000 generations previous to modern men and women. What would their health be like? Would they suffer from heart disease, diabetes, cancer, or dementia? How long would they live? The TRUTH is they did not suffer from those illnesses and would thrive to an old age. We know this to be true for many reasons. First, it just makes common sense diseases with known causes, such as tobacco, sugar, pesticides, and chemicals, did not exist. People did not die from heart disease and cancer, they died from trauma and infection. Second, people are still alive who live a Paleo lifestyle. Societies in the South Pacific, Eskimos, some parts of Africa, and Australian Aborigines grow old and are typically healthy. Bang and Dyerberg observed the Greenland Eskimos for 10 years and found not one death occurred from cardiovascular cause.[51] I mentored medical students who travelled into the jungles of the Philippines and lived with primitive cultures. They describe many elders who were active members of their society. Third, explorers from Captain Cook to Columbus and Magellan document cultures from around the world as healthy and thriving without the illnesses of more "civilized" societies.

★**LIVE WELL**: As the world changed from hunter-gatherers to farmers to industrialization, nutrition has changed as well, and not for the better.

Weston A. Price, a dentist who travelled by boat with his wife in the 1920's, described "Paleo" life and health in an amazing book called *Nutrition and Physical Degeneration*. He found the men stood straight and tall without decayed or overcrowded teeth. He found little evidence of the diseases so rampant today. Fast-forward to the present, where every child needs braces because their rotting teeth are crammed in a small mouth. This is a consequence of the child eating sugar and the nutrition (or lack thereof) of the mother while the child was in utero.

Where did the human race go wrong? The answer lies with the conversion from hunter-gatherer to agriculture-based nutrition. Researchers such as Boyd Eaton, Loren Cordain, and Laura Johnson-Kelly document this transition in peer-reviewed studies, lectures, and books. The universal theme from these scientists is that agriculture led to gastrointestinal disorders. Once the gut is damaged, every ailment with the longest of labels will arise. Vitamins and minerals become deficient. Inflammation and autoimmune disease become rampant. Cardiovascular damage, cancer, arthritis, and brain disorders are the end results.

What was once an active life, hunting and gathering, became sedentary. Instead of exerting energy to get your meal, you could sit around and wait for someone else to do it. The blacksmith, the cobbler, and the baker sat in the shop all day, eating grain-based foods. Obesity would shortly follow in addition to every other possible malady. Animals were cruelly corralled and their milk was used for a large portion of the new human diet. Never mind cow's milk is for baby cows as giraffe's milk is for baby giraffes. Once humans found sugar, the medical problems skyrocketed.

★**LIVE WELL**: Agriculture-based nutrition—grain, dairy products, and sugar—is the real culprit behind most diseases today.

So disease spirals out of control in the early 1900's and even the brightest of minds are left wondering why. As above, it seemed so easy to understand that grain, dairy, and sugar were the cause. Gary Taubes in *Good Calories, Bad Calories*, provides a chronicled modern dietary history. Taubes tells the story of William Banting, who published his own weight loss success in the 1860s, following what is clearly a Paleo-type diet. Around the same time, many others promoted nutrition guidelines all sharing the theme of carbohydrate restriction. Most of the research came from patients who were noted to have diabetes. This blood sugar disorder was quickly correlated with sugar, grain, and starch consumption. The treatment by avoidance was obvious and highly successful.

In the 1950's, coronary artery disease became front-page news. President Eisenhower suffered a heart attack and became saddled with recurrent chest pain called angina. The villains were falsely determined to be fat and cholesterol because they were found at the scene of the crime—autopsy evidence in heart vessels (this is like saying fireman caused the fire). Led by Ancil Keys, dietary guidelines focused on the prevention of heart disease by avoiding fat and cholesterol. Keys published data from seven countries, concluding those with the highest fat intake had the highest incidence of coronary disease. He conveniently did not include France and Switzerland; both consume a high fat diet, yet have a low incidence of heart disease. That was a "key" error (get it, key error, Ancil Keys).

★LIVE WELL: In the 1950s, heart disease was falsely associated with high levels of fat intake and cholesterol in the body.

The so-called French Paradox is not a paradox at all. The French invalidate the conclusion that fat causes heart disease, as they have a low incidence of heart problems, yet eat a high percentage of fat. Had Keys included 22 countries with existing data on fat intake and heart disease, his study would yield a different outcome, notably dietary fat is not associated with heart disease. A meta-analysis on over 300,000 patients, published in the *American Journal of Clinical Nutrition*, confirms saturated fat has no association with heart disease.[52] But the damage from Keys was done. He was included on a task force to revise dietary guidelines, which ultimately promoted a low fat diet. To top it off, Senator George McGovern waged war on dietary fat and led a massive change in government policy in the 1970's. The obesity cure with low carbohydrate intake was well known, but McGovern jumped on the anti-fat/anti-cholesterol bandwagon. The low fat/low cholesterol plan promoted by Keys and McGovern is a dismal failure for all medical conditions, as is evidenced by the continued explosion of obesity and disease.

★LIVE WELL: Saturated fat does not cause heart disease.

Doctors who promote a vegan diet are experimenting on their patients. In the history of the world, a vegan society never existed. All cultures ate meat and/or seafood. Gorillas and other primates are commonly used as an example of a vegan ancestor; however, people conveniently forget primates continuously eat insects. In fact, every wild animal would get their share of invertebrate critters mixed in with their veggies. Do you think a giraffe washes off the bugs prior to consuming leaves from a tree? Heck, there are even species of plants that eat insects!

Vegan cheerleaders point to studies that conclude a diet void of animal products lowers cholesterol. Cholesterol reduction is not something I would want, as discussed in my chapter, "Cholesterol is King." Remember, everyone has a perfect Paleo lipid profile genetically designed for them. Those who strictly reduce fat intake may indeed lower cholesterol. The reason is, they are not giving the body the tools it needs to make cholesterol and other life sustaining molecules. Blood levels also drop because the cholesterol typically manufactured for digestion becomes unnecessary. If you do not eat fat, you do not need as much bile cholesterol. Lastly, since the body is not making much cholesterol, the cells that are starving for it will clear LDL from the blood stream. Once again, if you do not eat animal fat, you are starving the body of essential nutrition.

★**LIVE WELL**: Every animal eats meat and/or insects. Some plants eat bugs!

Don't get me wrong, I love eating vegetables and the green leaf variety are the foundation of a healthy diet. In no way do I advocate eating meat and seafood 24/7 (although the Eskimos and tribes in Africa do and enjoy fantastic health). In fact, I think going raw vegan is an excellent short-term cleanse for our bodies. I juice fast twice a year. But let's face facts. The vegan diet is not complete. Vegan food combinations are an unsuccessful attempt to equal animal protein content. So many vegans eventually give up this diet when their stores of essential nutrients run out. They feel fatigued, lose muscle tone, and complain of a brain fog similar to dementia. Vegans and vegetarians of Indian heritage have the worst coronary disease. For an excellent read from a recovering vegan, check out *The Vegetarian Myth* by Lierre Kieth.

Why do doctors rarely talk about nutrition with their patients? For one, we are not trained in nutrition. Number two, most doctors eat the same crap as their patients. Trust me, I saw the garbage most M.D.'s shoved into their mouths. Why would they waste time talking to you about food when they cannot control themselves? My former group had fat cardiologists, some of which would be classified as obese.

Let's take a look at the foods that are definitely not Paleo, and definitely not healthy.

SUGAR

There is little doubt sugar is the absolute worst food for your health. Except for the Chocolate Cookie Diet, all experts agree sugar is poison. Unfortunately, sugar is the most addictive food on the planet and is responsible for more deaths than all drugs, pharmaceutical and illegal, combined. A recent report found as much as 25% of the American population's calorie consumption is from added sugar! I guess this is not surprising given the amount of soda, ice cream, cereal, and candy consumed. These totals do not include fruit, grain, and dairy products, which are all quickly digested into sugar.

> ★**LIVE WELL**: The worst food you can put into your body is sugar, and you are probably doing it in large amounts every day.

Sugar comes in many different forms and is usually hidden on labels to trick the consumer, if they even read the label. High fructose corn syrup, fructose, sucrose, corn syrup, agave nectar, fruit juice concentrate, evaporated cane juice, brown rice syrup, and anything else ending in "ose" is sugar incognito. Read the carbohydrate and sugar content of all packaged goods. Check the amount of servings in the container, as one serving of cereal may only contain 5 grams of sugar, but the serving size is 1/3 of a cup. Who eats 1/3 of a cup of cereal? I used to eat the whole box.

There are many forces who deny sugar is bad for our health. Organizations like The American Sugar Alliance and The Sugar Association have their agenda, as do Kellogg's, Nabisco, and General Mills. These groups fight the truth with bogus studies and information while spending millions of dollars on false advertising and lining the pockets of national decision makers like the USDA. Quitting sugar is not easy and the world is against us. Conquering this demon is a physical and emotional battle. But trust me, it can be done, and you can do it. I say this because there is no bigger sugar addict than myself, but I slayed the beast and so have hundreds of my patients. This isn't to say you can never eat sugar again, but once per week should be the maximum. A weekly treat should only be consumed after you hit your goal weight.

★**LIVE WELL**: Your addiction to sugar can be conquered, but corporate America is against you.

Just recently, a large trial was completed that proved the obvious: sugar causes cardiovascular disease. In fact, those people who ate the most sugar faced an increased death rate of 250%.[53] The well-known researcher and pediatric endocrinologist Robert Lusting released a study in 2013 showing that for every additional 150kcal of sugar daily (one can of soda), diabetes risk increases by 1%. This data is exciting because the American Diabetes Association (ADA) are deniers of the fact sugar increases diabetes risk, pinning diabetes on obesity itself. Without people eating sugar, diabetes will go bye-bye and so will the jobs at the ADA. Remember the quote by Upton Sinclair, "It is hard to get a person to understand something when his job depends on not understanding it." The ADA is highly funded by "Big Sugar." The human body did not evolve with this massive sugar onslaught in mind.

★**LIVE WELL**: You CANNOT get fat without eating sugar and grain.

By now, most people know the ramifications of becoming diabetic. Diabetes affects millions of people and conjures up images of insulin shots, dialysis due to kidney failure, and even amputated limbs. The reality is most diabetics will not suffer from those conditions. What diabetes DOES is put you at an increased risk for just about everything from heart disease to dementia to cancer. But diabetes is only a label for those who meet a certain blood sugar level. Any amount of blood sugar above normal will increase your risk, and fasting blood sugar should be less than 85.

Studies show diabetics are at a three-fold risk of heart disease, cancer, and dementia.[54] If you are labeled with pre-diabetes, your risk of dying from heart disease is 60% higher.[55] Insulin is a hormone released by the pancreas that controls blood sugar storage in addition to fat and protein control. An elevated fasting insulin level increases CV risk by 30%.[56] Fasting insulin is easy to test for and should be a part of any blood work to assess cardiovascular, cancer, and dementia risk.

★LIVE WELL: Diabetes leads to triple the risk of heart disease, cancer, and dementia.

Meat, seafood, nuts, seeds, and eggs do not raise blood sugar. I challenge my diabetes patients to drink a glass of olive oil or eat a half-dozen eggs and see what happens with their blood sugar. It barely moves. Eat a slice of whole wheat bread and watch blood sugar skyrocket. Carbohydrates are quickly broken down into glucose, galactose, and fructose, which consequently raise blood glucose. This glucose leads to the AGEing of the body. Here AGE stands for advanced glycosylated end-products, which damage cellular and protein structures. Starch from grains, potatoes, and beans are broken down into glucose that is quickly absorbed, leading to an insulin spike. Sugar is the best way to get fat and, like drugs, is extremely addictive. Just watch a child on the hunt for sugar. Hemoglobin A1C is a common way to test for the AGEing of the body.

★LIVE WELL: Grains, potatoes, and beans are starches that turn into glucose. Sugar highs are highly addictive!

Chocolate is often touted as a health food. It is true the cacao bean, the main ingredient in this treat, has some significant antioxidant properties and is loaded with vitamins and minerals. But chocolate is packed with sugar, dairy, and other unhealthy items. Even dark chocolate often contains a significant amount of sugar. Raw cacao has a bitter taste, which most people do not like. It also contains theobromine, a compound similar to caffeine, causing symptoms of palpitations and anxiety in many people.

The myriad of symptoms from sugar creates a long list. One of the first books I read was *Sugar Shock* by Connie Bennett. Here Connie describes how anxiety, depression, and dozens of other complaints are related to sugar intake. For example, my patient Janice, age 42, felt palpitations for years that completely resolved after one week without sugar. Another example is Chad, age 27, with frequent lightheadedness, who was cured with a low sugar diet. A sugar-free diet has worked to resolve non-cardiac chest pain that was likely muscular in origin.

★**LIVE WELL**: Any of your complaints can be caused by sugar.

GRAIN

Wheat, barley, rye, oats, corn, etc. are grains that need to be heavily processed to allow for human consumption. These items are a recent addition to the human diet and lead to many medical ailments. Grains are heavily promoted by corporations because they are cheap to manufacture and boast a long shelf life. Companies like Nabisco and Kellogg's hold all the money, therefore they control the politicians and the guidelines. Accordingly, the moronic Food Pyramid recommends we all consume 6-11 servings of grain per day. This is not based on science or health, but solely on money. The fact General Mills can claim Cheerios is heart-healthy is a travesty and should rock the foundation of the food pyramid. The product label claims this particular cereal lowers cholesterol by 4%. Who cares? Does it lower cardiac risk? A surgeon can remove your liver and your cholesterol will drop by 75%. Chemotherapy lowers cholesterol. You can eat a cardboard box and lower cholesterol. It tastes the same as unsweetened Cheerios. Speaking of cereal, check out the advertising for Raisin Bran. This product touts heart health, yet contains 20 grams of sugar per serving. Who is policing these corporations from filling the airwaves with lies to trick the American public?

★**LIVE WELL**: Beware—cereals are not heart-healthy, despite the advertising.

GLUTEN

Gluten, a nasty protein found in many grains, destroys the gastrointestinal lining, often resulting in Celiac disease. Celiac patients must avoid even minute amounts of gluten or suffer from bloody bowel movements and severe abdominal pain. It is estimated that 50-70% of the population is gluten intolerant. Gluten has been linked to coronary disease, arthritic conditions, cancer, diabetes, and thyroid disease. You name the symptoms, gluten is likely the cause. Astute doctors recommend avoiding wheat, barley, and rye, but patients switch to other "carbolicious" grains that are gluten-free. This situation is not much better. Gluten-free is still full of carbohydrates and can irritate the gut, and hence the rest of the body. In fact, the Cyrex Corporation runs a blood panel on grains that induce a gluten-like sensitivity. Gluten-free products often contain more sugar to make up for taste, and other additives to get the texture of bread, pasta, and other baked goods. These additives are not healthy and may be from corn and soy. Gluten-free is rarely organic. Is it possible coronary artery disease is caused by gluten? The answer is obvious.

★**LIVE WELL**: Gluten is bad for you, but "gluten-free" may not be much better.

The *No Grain Diet* by Joseph Mercola, D.O., and *Going Against The Grain* by Melissa Smith are excellent reads for more information. *Grain Brain* by neurologist David Perlmutter, M.D., was recently published and has been on the best-seller list. He documents the damage grain causes to the brain, including dementia and other neurodegenerative diseases. Another great read is *Wheat Belly* by William Davis, M.D. He chronicles the changes in our health that go along with the modification of wheat since biblical days. The medical establishment is way behind on this issue.

DAIRY

Do you suffer from sinus congestion, allergies, or asthma? The first things to get rid of are dairy products. Bowel issues, such as heartburn, diarrhea, gas, or bloating, are often caused by milk. Cow milk is for baby cows, monkey milk is for baby monkeys, and human milk is for baby humans. Our ancestors did not chase after other animals to milk them and create butter, cheese, yogurt, and ice cream. Our bodies are not genetically programmed to consume animal milk, and it does not do a body good. No science exists to support the relationship between milk and bone health. The United States is one of the biggest consumers of dairy products, yet it has the highest incidence of osteoporosis. Cows don't drink milk and their bones are just fine. We get osteoporosis from non-Paleo foods, chemicals, and lack of exercise.

★**LIVE WELL**: The connection between milk and good bone health is another medical myth.

Casein is a protein found in milk, cheese, and yogurt. Butter and cream tend to contain lower levels of casein. This protein is a cause of irritation and, in my experience, shows up as a problem on food sensitivity panels about 25% of the time. Ghee, or clarified butter, is free of casein and may be safe to consume. Always read food labels because milk-derived ingredients, such as whey, protein powder, powdered milk, artificial butter flavor and artificial cheese flavor, can contain small amounts of casein. Whey is an excellent source of protein in the powdered form as long as you are not part of the 25% who are sensitive to it. Whey builds glutathione, the main anti-oxidant of the body. If you are looking for an excellent source of protein as a supplement, check out beef protein.

★**LIVE WELL**: Ghee and whey are two beneficial dairy products, but only if you are not already sensitive to milk products.

We are born with the digestive enzyme lactase. Most people lose this enzyme in late childhood because historically the body no longer needs it after we stop nursing. Milk contains lactose, which is milk sugar that increases diabetes rates and heart disease risk. Name the gastrointestinal symptom and lactose intolerance is at the top of the list of causes.

If you are going to consume milk, the most natural way would be in its raw state. That way, you are getting milk the way nature intended, full of fat, cholesterol, and vitamins. Raw milk is live, meaning it contains enzymes that assist with digestion and contain healthy probiotics. Processed milk is pasteurized and homogenized into a form no animal can recognize as food. All of the nutrition is stripped in processing, and a cheap multivitamin is added back. If you consume dairy, make sure you take digestive enzymes prior to eating or drinking.

★**LIVE WELL**: If you drink milk, do it raw.

SOY

I often quote Kayla Daniel to my patients whenever I discuss nutrition. She is a Ph.D. and nutritionist who wrote *The Whole Soy Story*. This book destroys the soy argument in less than 500 pages. Bottom line, our Paleo ancestors never ate soy, certainly not in the form of tofu or soy bacon. To feed an infant soy milk and then state it is equivalent to human breast milk is a crime. Soy became huge in the 1970s based on spurious claims by aggressive marketers. Advertising campaigns pulled at our heartstrings with claims soy could solve world hunger. The public was told to stay away from saturated fats like coconut oil because it causes heart disease. How convenient for candy companies and other food manufacturers to replace expensive coconut from the South Pacific with cheap soybean oil from the Midwest. Soybean oil is a mere fraction of the cost of coconut oil. References to Asian diets and longevity lead us to believe that soy is the fountain of youth. First, Asians do not live much longer than the sickly US population. Second, according to K.C. Chang in *Food in Chinese Culture*, Asians consume small amounts of mostly fermented soy. The majority of calories in the Chinese diet are from meat and seafood. Tell that to well published vegans T. Colin Campbell, author of the *China Study*, and to Dr. Esselstyn and his son, who wrote *Engine Number 2*.

> ★LIVE WELL: The majority of calories in the Asian diet are from meat and seafood.

PESTICIDES

Plain and simple . . . you MUST EAT ORGANIC FOOD. If pesticides kill bugs, they will kill us. It may take a little more time, but the chemical poisons will do damage. Our health is suffering and the planet is quickly under destruction. One study demonstrated that farmers who apply pesticides suffer from an increase in heart attacks and deaths.[57] A study from 2012 found a much higher risk of carotid atherosclerosis in those people with the highest levels of POP's (persistent organic pollutants).[58] The carotids are the arteries that supply the brain, so they are pretty important to most people. The more disease in the carotid arteries, the higher your risk of stroke. Blood levels of POP's can be tested by various companies, including Genova Diagnostics.

The Monsanto corporation has been "kind" enough to give the world Round-Up herbicide. This chemical is heavily sprayed on crops genetically engineered to be resistant to its effects. Everything else dies, but the soy lives. Round-Up is sprayed at schools, athletic fields, and just about every other square inch of earth. Round-Up contains a variety of toxins, but the worst is likely glyphosate. Studies find that glyphosate:[59]

1. Increases lipid peroxidation (damages LDL)
2. Increases blood stickiness
3. Damages the vascular endothelium
4. Blocks mineral absorption
5. Increases ammonia (brain fog)
6. Decreases amino acid production
7. Increases risk of dangerous gut bacterial infections
8. Leads to formaldehyde production (cancer and brain disease)

When it comes to pesticides, the list of health ramifications is long and includes:[60]

- Dementia
- Parkinson's disease- over 65 studies
- Cancer- over 100 studies
- Diabetes
- Hormonal abnormalities
- Asthma
- Birth defects- 22 studies
- Heart disease

Are there skeptics in your life regarding the benefits of eating organic foods? There are hundreds of studies about pesticides on produce, including a recent 2014 article finding organic food has more antioxidants and less cadmium. All this in addition to a quarter of the pesticide residues.[61]

★LIVE WELL: Once in your body, pesticides are a no-brainer—literally.

ARTIFICIAL INGREDIENTS

Everyone tries to cheat the system. In other words, people want the thrill of eating sweet foods, but they also want to avoid the calories or negative health ramifications that come with such foods. Unfortunately, it is not that easy.

Artificial sweeteners, like aspartame, acesulfame, and sucralose are not part of a healthy diet and lifestyle. These products trick the body into thinking something sweet is coming its way. There is no proof they lead to any meaningful weight loss. In fact, as the consumption of artificial sweeteners has increased, so has the incidence of obesity.[62] Studies show double the risk of diabetes and lipid abnormalities in those who consumed the most artificially sweetened beverages.[63] Diabetes may be the number one risk factor for coronary artery disease! Speaking of coronary artery disease, in a study of over 88,000 nurses, artificial sweeteners were associated with a higher risk of heart attacks, stroke, and death.[64]

★**LIVE WELL**: Artificial sweeteners play a double trick on your body: they taste sweet without any calories, but they increase your chance of heart disease, diabetes, and obesity.

Let's take a look at aspartame, sold under brand names like NutraSweet and Equal, and found in many diet soft drinks. This unnatural substance is comprised of phenylalanine, aspartic acid, and methanol. Phenylalanine is an amino acid precursor to the neurotransmitters dopamine, norepinephrine, and epinephrine in the body. These are potent constrictors of blood vessels. Could this lead to hypertension? Those same neurotransmitters can stimulate the heart leading to tachycardia (fast heart rate) and rhythm disorders such as atrial fibrillation or worse. In fact, an article from 2009 found aspartame and monosodium glutamate (MSG) increase the risk of atrial fibrillation.[65]

Aspartic acid consumption has been linked with strokes, seizures, dementia, and Parkinson's disease. Methanol or wood alcohol breaks down into formaldehyde, which the EPA considers a carcinogen (cancer-causing agent). One can of diet soda contains 2x the FDA limit on safe consumption of methanol.

★**LIVE WELL**: The effects of NutraSweet and Equal are not so sweet for your body.

Water treatment facilities do not break down most artificial sweeteners,[66] so they remain in the water supply. Make sure you drink clean water. Artificial sweeteners go into breast milk and can affect babies. They stimulate fat cells to get fatter and suppress fat breakdown. They cause genetic damage.[67]

Stevia comes from a leaf. There are some positive studies using the actual leaf, but this is not what is sold in stores or in pre-packaged goods. What is sold is a chemically tainted derivative more likely harmful than helpful. Two of my patients with acne got resolution of their skin condition after giving up Stevia. Just be careful using this product; if you enjoy it, grow your own.

Bottom line—stay natural. Use raw honey or maple syrup if you need to add a little sweetness to your life. These are Paleo foods that were available to our ancestors. Herbal tea and sparking water are great tools to fight sugar cravings. Or do what I do—mix up a greens drink. I will share more about this with you in Chapter 16.

★**LIVE WELL**: Use natural sweeteners, like honey and maple syrup, or grow your own stevia plants.

MSG stands for monosodium glutamate. Much has been written about this maligned molecule. Over the years, I found many patients to be sensitive to this food additive. Read the labels for hidden MSG as hydrolyzed vegetable protein, yeast extract, soy extract, or protein isolates. Name the symptoms and MSG can be the cause. Cardiovascular effects of MSG are well documented.[68]

The intake of MSG leads to:

1.   Damaged blood vessels
2.   Reduced antioxidant production
3.   Increased oxidative stress
4.   Damaged LDL particles
5.   Increased blood clotting
6.   Insulin resistance
7.   Atrial fibrillation

Watch out for artificial colors with names like Blue Lake 40 and Red 6. The body does not recognize these toxins and will react negatively. There is plenty of data linking these petroleum-based food additives to psychiatric issues and cancer. Blue dye number 1 and 2 are linked with cancer in animal tests, while red dye number 3 causes thyroid tumors in rats. Green dye number 3 is linked to bladder cancer, and yellow dye number 6 is linked to tumors of the kidneys and adrenal glands. Although intriguing, do we need a study to tell us artificial petroleum-based products are bad for the heart and vessels? There are natural ways to color food and make tasty natural treats by using beets, wheat grass, and berry juices.

★**LIVE WELL**: One pet-peeve is when people say moderation is the key. Moderation is NOT the key. Moderation will kill you.

CASE STUDY

Judy was a 53-year-old female who complained of fatigue, diarrhea, and dark circles under her eyes. She thought her face looked 20 years older than her actual age. She came to my office looking for the magic supplement. "It does not exist," I told her. But, I explained, what does work is good nutrition, chemical avoidance, detox, and supplements. Reluctantly, she started to follow Paleo and began nutrients to heal her gut. Within two months, she returned to my office with a big smile on her face and no dark circles. The diarrhea was gone and her energy returned. Since then, Judy has referred at least ten patients to my practice.

ACTION PLAN

Foods to Avoid:

1. Sugar
2. Artificial colors, flavor, and sweeteners
3. Wheat and gluten containing grains
4. Soy
5. Corn
6. Dairy such as milk, cheese, butter, yogurt, and cream

Foods to limit:

1. Grains such as rice, buckwheat, millet, sorghum, amaranth, quinoa
2. Beans
3. Fruit
4. Potatoes
5. Nightshades such as eggplant, peppers, and tomatoes

No matter what diet you follow, please use these simple rules:

1. Eat organic and definitely no GMO (genetically modified foods).
2. Eat plenty of organic vegetables with every meal.
3. Avoid sugar.
4. Chew your food well.
5. No electronics at the table. Make meals a time of relaxation and conversation.
6. Eat two-thirds raw to one-third cooked food.
7. Avoid all artificial colors, flavors, and sweeteners.
8. Limit fluid around meals to concentrate your gastric enzymes.
9. Eat at home where food can be prepared healthy, and it's cheaper too.
10. You may benefit from digestive enzymes and betaine HCL at the beginning of meals. More on this in Chapter 16.

Chapter 5

ONE NATION UNDER PROZAC

"Laughter is the Best Medicine."
—Unknown

F or years, I have educated my patients on the two things that cause all disease: poor nutrition and chemicals. But over time I came to realize physical inactivity, lack of quality sleep, and mental disorders may be equally as important. I know the label 'mental disorders' brings Jack Nicholson to mind in "The Shining" and "One Flew Over the Cuckoos Nest," but they aren't always that extreme. Mental disorders include stress, depression, anxiety, anger, and social isolation. It is not a secret that in today's society of information overload, political turmoil, and financial unrest, the health of America is suffering. Some amount of mental distress is normal and probably healthy. Our ancestors no doubt had some of the same feelings. But clearly the problem is worsening. The American Psychological Association (APA) found 80% of respondents reported an increase in stress over only one year.[69] The fact is, the rise of cardiovascular disease parallels the increase in mental health disorders.

During my ten years of medical training, I cannot recall ever discussing mental disorders and their relation to physical health. Even on my psychiatry rotation as a third year student, the focus was on medications. Mental problems, and how to deal with them, are rarely discussed in the short office visit with a primary care doctor. If the subject comes up, going after the cause is not likely— the pharmaceutical approach is always first in line. One nation under Prozac has to stop.

Poor Nutrition

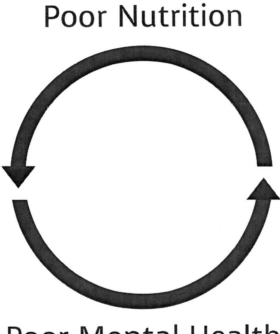

Poor Mental Health

In a bizarre circle, poor mental health often leads to bad food, alcohol, drugs (prescription and over-the-counter), tobacco, little exercise, and numerous other unhealthy lifestyle choices. All of these factors alter the gut microbiome, the bacteria crucial for health. Many studies conclude the variety of probiotics in your intestines influences mental health.[70] Lousy nutrition clearly contributes to poor mental health. Eating sugar and fast food cannot prepare you for the rigors of life as effectively as an organic, Paleo diet. Gluten, for example, destroys the intestinal barrier; therefore, nutrients are not absorbed and inflammation is rampant. Some of those critical nutrients include B12 and fatty acids, both vital for brain health. Omega-3 fat from seafood is necessary for our brain. There is exciting research using probiotics to improve mental health.[71]

★**LIVE WELL**: Poor nutrition and poor mental health go hand in hand.

Could poor mental and physical health actually start in the womb or even before conception? So many young women eat junk food, ingest pharmaceuticals like ibuprofen and psych meds, and are drowning in chemicals. Because of this toxic burden, the developing mind of a child has little chance. Sadly, many children are not breast fed, which increases the risk of mental health problems. Additionally, children are given antibiotics for the slightest fever, leading to a loss of healthy gut bacteria. Then, when the child acts out at the age of 5, drugs are prescribed and a lifetime of pharmaceuticals begins.

There are five major areas to address regarding mental health: stress, depression, anxiety, anger, and social isolation. We will discuss these feelings and an action plan to resolve them. Certainly, if you feel overburdened and this chapter really rings home to you, seek out professional help (not a pill-pushing psychiatrist) so you can work through these issues in a natural fashion. Drugs only cover up symptoms and do not get to the cause of disease. There is no data suggesting psychiatric drugs decrease cardiovascular events.

★**LIVE WELL**: Mental health starts in the womb.

STRESS—WHAT WE THINK CAN BECOME REALITY

Most of us would consider ourselves to be under stress, but what does that word really mean? Stress refers to both physical and emotional challenges, some of which may be transient and rather harmless such as short-duration exercise, test taking, or a work deadline. These scenarios may be positive and are considered similar to our caveman brethren who ran after food, and ran away from becoming food. Dealing with Mother Nature was usually not a difficult task and most likely our ancestors led a relatively peaceful existence. But modern stress may be chronic and uncontrollable (e.g., caregiving for a loved one with a terminal illness, financial issues, relationship problems), leading to body dysfunction and ultimately symptomatic disease. Searching the words "stress" and "coronary artery disease" reveals over 17,000 studies on the health journal site PubMed. Does the body truly have a negative response to stress, or are the real issues poor nutrition and lifestyle choices? The answer lies in the multitude of studies done on animals in a controlled environment, which clearly demonstrate stress by itself leads to adverse health consequences.

Unsurprisingly, there are well-established connections between stress and cardiovascular disease. A study from 2002 looked at men and women correlating stress with metabolic syndrome (MetS) and heart disease. MetS is the group of findings, including hypertension, obesity, abnormal lipids, and elevated blood sugar, associated with a marked increase in cardiovascular problems. The authors found that caregiver men (those taking care of another person) had twice the risk of heart disease compared to non-caregiver men. The women caregivers with sleep issues, distress, anger, and hostility also had worse outcomes.[72] The MetS association is not surprising, given the fact data shows increased blood sugar and fasting insulin levels in those with perceived stress. These are significant predictors of heart and neurologic issues. Markers of inflammation rise during acute stress.[73]

★**LIVE WELL**: Stress is more than merely job-related; poor nutrition and lifestyle choices create stress and increase the risk of heart problems.

Heart attacks are 50% more common in those complaining of stress versus those who don't. Survival from a heart attack is lower in those individuals experiencing high stress. In one eye-opening investigation, Milani and Lavie found patients with high psychosocial stress in cardiac rehabilitation were almost four times as likely to die as those with low stress.[74]. Caretakers of people with chronic health conditions maintain higher resting heart rates, higher blood pressure, and a greater incidence of the metabolic syndrome. Inflammation markers are also higher. A recent report found the loss of a spouse doubles the risk of a heart attack or stroke in the following 30 days.[75] There are many stressful categories in a Life Event Scale and all are likely to increase the risk of cardiovascular events. This ranges from getting married to getting divorced, losing a job to getting a promotion. Job stress is reported to increase the risk of a cardiac event by four-fold;[76] it also increases the risk of carotid atherosclerosis.[77] One study found that subjecting coronary disease patients to mental stress actually made their heart function worse.[78]

It is well known Monday mornings and return from a vacation or holiday are popular times to suffer a heart attack. I saw these scenarios play out for many years. The morning after Daylight Savings time in the spring leads to more cardiac events (more on this in Chapter 11). Heart attacks are more common during the Super Bowl.[79] One thing I noted was a rise in hospital admissions after basketball playoff games in Chicago. Watching Michael Jordan and the Bulls in the 90's make their run for another title proved too much for some people.

A scary trend over the last ten years is the rise of Takotsubo syndrome, also known as "Broken Heart Syndrome." In this scenario, a stressful event leads to a heart attack and damaged heart muscle. When an angiogram is performed, no blockage is found. An artery spasm from an epinephrine surge is the likely culprit. This was a rare diagnosis during my training, but it appears to be on a rapid rise. Middle-aged women are the most frequent victims.

★LIVE WELL: No matter the source, stress can lead to high blood pressure, heart attack, and even death.

DEPRESSION

The more depressed you are, the higher your risk of cardiovascular disease. In one study, an affirmative answer to the question "[During the last month] have you felt so sad, discouraged, hopeless, or had so many problems that you wondered if anything was worthwhile?" more than doubled the risk of heart disease. Men who experience hopelessness develop significantly more carotid atherosclerosis over time.[80] Those with depression have enhanced platelet reactivity and are more likely to form blood clots. Stress hormones, such as cortisol and adrenaline, are elevated in those who are depressed. Reduced heart rate variability in stressed-out people is a dangerous sign associated with heart problems. Depressed patients may be more prone to heart artery spasm.[81] In animal studies the endothelium, which lines every major artery, is dysfunctional when stress is present.

★**LIVE WELL**: Depression, like stress, can increase the risk of a cardiac event.

As we age, the chaotic heart rhythm known as atrial fibrillation is more common. I successfully utilize natural approaches to this condition, whereas drugs and electrical cardioversion are typically used by mainstream cardiologists. Interestingly, depressed patients are more likely to revert to atrial fibrillation after successful cardioversion.[82] Trust me, you do not want to undergo this procedure more than once. Your doctor needs to address these issues prior to cardioversion. How often is this discussed? Never.

ANXIETY

Anxiety is one of the most prevalent psychiatric disorders in the general population with over 50% of people fitting the criteria. Some level of anxiety may be normal, but when it turns into abnormal behavior, such as pacing back and forth or binge eating, it crosses the line. People with high levels of anxiety often admit to physical complaints, such as chest pain, shortness of breath, and bowel issues. For many patients with chest pain that is clearly not caused by their heart, the symptoms are most likely anxiety. This diagnosis should be on the bottom of a doctor's list as we assess for more life-threatening medical conditions; but nonetheless, anxiety is one of the most common causes of chest pain. But the scary reality is anxiety can clearly provoke a heart event.

In a study of 1,457 white men, aged 40-64, anxiety was strongly related to subsequent heart disease. In fact, those with the highest amounts of self-reported anxiety had almost four times the risk of cardiovascular events. The more anxiety, the higher the risk.[83] In 1988, a survey was conducted of 33,999 American male health professionals who were free from cardiovascular disease at baseline. Levels of anxiety were assessed and the men were followed for future cardiac events. This study showed the risk to be three times greater among those with the worst anxiety![84] A study published in the journal Circulation had similar findings.[85] A separate study revealed extra heartbeats, known as PVC's, were more common in anxious individuals.

★**LIVE WELL**: Anxiety leads to heart attacks and irregular heartbeats.

What is it about anxiety that causes an increase in cardiovascular events such as sudden death and heart attacks? The authors from the above studies proposed a couple of ideas. One issue appears to be a catecholamine (adrenaline) surge leading to an abnormal heart rhythm. Another explanation is that a coronary spasm, in which one of the heart arteries suddenly closes down leading to heart damage, is precipitated by anxiety-induced hyperventilation. Anxiety may also lead to unhealthy diet choices such as sugar, caffeine, and other non-Paleo foods.

Years ago while I was a medical resident, a good friend of mine and I were heading out on a Saturday night in downtown Chicago. After a long week at the hospital and a brutal night on call, I was ready for a good time. My friend was under a lot of stress from his job and some family matters. The stress clearly manifested itself that night into significant anxiety on his part. He did not feel well from the start, then complained of numbness in his left arm. His concern led us to the emergency room instead of the planned restaurant. When he was seen by the triage nurse who checked his vital signs, even I was shocked to learn his blood pressure was 240/120. After three days of testing, my buddy was sent home with a prescription for Valium. I, however, was left with an important lesson about the power of anxiety and stress. These factors are not to be taken lightly.

★**LIVE WELL**: Anxiety can produce an adrenaline surge, which can lead to an abnormal heart rhythm.

ANGER

Anger and hostility bring to mind a cartoon of a flush-faced character ready to blow his top off. The actual medical consequences of anger are not far off. We all need to release some steam once in a while and drop a few four-letter words, but doing this repetitively is clearly unhealthy. Search anger and cardiovascular on pubmed.gov (the government database of medical literature) and over 670 articles come up. This is a major problem.

Multiple studies find anger increases the risk of suffering a heart attack and sudden cardiac death.[86] Many times I consulted on a heart attack victim whose event was brought on by an argument with a family member or intolerable boss. Anger can lead to adrenal and cortisol surges, which in turn leads to plaque rupture and coronary artery spasm. Anger also leads to the blood becoming sticky or hypercoagulable. A study from 2011 found men with hostility had double the risk of cardiac events, such as heart attacks and strokes.[87]

★**LIVE WELL**: A recent study found marriage lowers heart attack risk.[88]

It is not surprising a psychiatric journal reported anger increases the risk of hypertension.[89] One of the mechanisms of high blood pressure in angry people may be related to the way blood vessels expand and contract. Anger clearly leads to an adrenaline surge, which raises blood pressure.[90] Interestingly, anger increases the risk of atrial fibrillation.[91] How many doctors do you think are asking patients about anger when it comes to controlling atrial fibrillation? My guess is the answer is zero. Disease of the carotid arteries, which supply the brain, is a major risk factor for having a stroke and is more commonly found in angry people.[92] Lastly, the recurrence of a blocked artery following an intervention is more common in angry people.[93] I think you are getting the point; anger is not good for our tickers.

★**LIVE WELL**: Anger increases the chance of hypertension, atrial fibrillation, and artery disease.

SOCIAL ISOLATION

Social relationships play a significant role in cardiovascular disease incidence, progression, and mortality. Social isolation is defined as having few close relationships or social ties in the community. Many people take for granted the benefits of family and good friends. I understand both are possible sources of stress, but the benefits of a good social network outweigh the bad. Social isolation unfortunately affects millions of people, especially seniors, but an alarming number of younger people are also feeling alone.

Many studies show feelings of loneliness raise the risk of cardiovascular events. A report from a medical journal found the risk of dying from cardiac cause was 2.5 times higher in those with three or fewer people in their social support group.[94] In the year following a heart attack, feeling isolated puts a person at the same death risk as classic cardiac risk factors like tobacco and diabetes. Multiple studies find the marker of inflammation called CRP is the highest in those with self-reported feelings of isolation. Not only is CRP linked to heart disease, but it is also associated with strokes and cancer.[95]

Social networking sites—most notably Facebook—are a powerful influence on how friendships are maintained in today's world. A continuously updated stream of information detailing the activities, thoughts, and feelings of friends enables a constant sense of connection. Some studies observe, in this sense, Facebook and related sites make it easier than ever to satisfy the need to belong. But other studies note this type of social interaction can also create opportunities for social rejection and bullying. In general, research weighing the psychological benefits and negative outcomes of this technology are mixed. Social Influence reported on a group of Facebook users divided into two groups: those who were allowed to post to Facebook and those not allowed. Isolation and depressive measures were clearly worse in those not allowed to post, and who thus lost the social interaction.

I do encourage all of my patients to follow and post on our Facebook page (shameless plug—facebook.com/thedrswolfson). This way, they can interact with us and get excellent information, realizing the ultimate goal of heart and total body health. In my years as a practicing medical doctor, I witnessed dozens of patients who had minimal contact with family or friends.

Many seniors do not drive, or endure physical limitations, keeping them from getting out of the house. This problem will grow as our population continues to age.

★**LIVE WELL**: Cultivate relationships in person, by phone, and through social media.

ACTION PLAN

The purpose of this chapter was to highlight the heart risks associated with mental health issues. Seek out professional help when necessary, but know that drugs are not the answer to social limitations, the loss of a spouse, or childhood trauma. How can you improve your mental health? I listed ten items here, but by no means is this list all-inclusive or comprehensive.

1. Eat healthy. It stands to reason people who eat the healthiest have less stress, and cope with stress better than fast food junkies. Give Paleo a try for a few weeks and see the benefits on your psyche.
2. Go meet your neighbors. Seek out healthy relationships. Join a club, get a hobby, or even go to the library. Do what it takes to find friendship in society. Your heart will benefit immensely.
3. Mend troublesome relationships or end them. Seek counseling if needed.
4. Exercise. According to Harvard Men's Health (and about a million other sources), exercise reduces stress. Exercise also lowers cardiac risk.
5. Take the right supplements. Evidence supports that vitamins C and D are stress relievers. Omega-3 fats, as documented in *The Omega-3 Connection*, produce a similar effect.
6. Get sunshine. The sun is the source of all life. Seasonal affective disorder is a type of depression, and sun exposure is the answer.
7. Practice relaxation techniques, yoga, tai chi, etc. One of my favorite smartphone apps is called Relax Lite from Saagara. I recommend it to all my patients and find those who do the program daily improve blood pressure.

8. Social media. This is a good way to engage with other people and cultivate relationships. Pen pals, email partners, and text messaging are excellent ways to stay in touch with people from afar.
9. Drink plenty of purified water.
10. Get thyroid, heavy metal, genetic, and nutrient testing.

Chapter 6

THE FAILED PROMISE
OF BIG PHARMA

*"The person who takes medicine for disease must recover twice,
once from the disease, and once from the medicine."*
—Sir William Osler

Americans spend trillions of dollars on billions of pharmaceutical prescriptions. In fact, drug manufacturers collected over $500 billion in revenue in 2013. For all of that money, you would think the health of Americans would be extraordinary. The reality is much different. Shockingly, life expectancy in the U.S. is 34th out of 35 industrialized countries, according to the Annual Review in Public Health.[96] In fact, our citizens die younger than people in Cuba and Costa Rica, despite the fact these are "developing" countries. Hopefully they are not developing our chronic diseases. In this chapter, we will discuss some of the biggest health issues within our society, and some of the medications Big Pharma promises will fix them. Amazingly, 90% of adults over age 60 take at least one prescription and 20% take over five different pills! The "pill for every ill" mentality must stop.

Despite pharmaceutical corporations essentially owning the medical schools and paying for most of the research in this country, drugs rarely make us live longer or better. Pharmaceuticals do not cure disease, just as surgery is never a cure. These are cover-ups and Band-Aid approaches. The factors leading to a sickly gall bladder are still present despite removal of the organ, just as the cause of breast cancer is still present in the woman despite a mastectomy. This kindergarten logic has never occurred to the vast majority of surgeons with the "cut to cure" mentality. Should our medical system be geared toward removing most of our organs to avoid sickness? How idiotic does that sound? My wife tells the story of her patient who, at 45, already had six organs removed (gall bladder, tonsils, appendix, uterus, ovaries, and thyroid). The patient confided in Heather how she wished to have met her before all the organs were cut out.

★**LIVE WELL**: 90% of adults over age 60 take at least one prescription. 20% take over five different pills.

Big Pharma sends in their fleet of models to wine and dine the docs, convincing them why a particular pharmaceutical should be prescribed. In fact, there are over 80,000 pharmaceutical representatives courting over 800,000 medical providers. The blatant payola today is not nearly as bad as in the '80s and '90s, yet Pharma still sponsors conferences and brings lunch to buy the love of docs. The reps almost make you feel guilty for not prescribing their drug, as if you would be committing malpractice. Actually, if you do not prescribe drugs in the guidelines produced by the medical elite, you could be found guilty of negligence. Who writes these guidelines? The doctors on the payroll of Big Pharma. Great system, huh?

New information comes out daily about the dangers of over-the-counter and prescription drugs. The Centers for Disease Control (CDC) estimates that over 750, 000 emergency room (ER) visits per year are for prescription adverse reactions.[97] The correct prescription for the correct person at the correct dose leads to hundreds of thousands of yearly ER visits. An unfortunate (but true) quip is that every drug pulled by the FDA because of safety reasons was once approved as safe by the FDA. Long-term studies are rarely done, certainly not prior to drug approval. In many cases, only after enough people die is the drug removed from the market. Do you ever see ads from attorneys looking for victims in giant class action lawsuits? These guys advertise 24/7 because people are adversely affected by drugs, and in some cases, die.

> ★LIVE WELL: A doctor prescribes a drug he knows little about, for a disease of which he knows even less, to a person of who he knows nothing. – **Source Unknown**

Recently, a group of drugs known as non-steroidal anti-inflammatories (NSAID's like ibuprofen) were found to increase the risk of atrial fibrillation by 76%.[98] Atrial fibrillation is a chaotic heart rhythm usually treated with pharmaceuticals or surgery. Patients are also put on blood thinners, which carry plenty of risk, as discussed later in this chapter. How many thousands went through an ablation procedure to burn heart tissue as a cure for AFIB, when the cause was ibuprofen?

Antibiotics are dispensed like candy to children and adults. There is rarely a true indication for these drugs, but doctors want to get patients out of the office quickly while attempting to make them happy. Usually patients come in with viral symptoms, looking for the cure through prescriptions. Antibiotics do not treat viruses! This overuse of an amazingly effective class of drugs has led to resistant bacteria. Doctors frequently reach for the newer and more expensive antibiotics, which will eventually render these drugs useless to soon-to-be resistant bacteria. All of this behavior stems from the fact that docs were catered with a free lunch. My father used to say, "Take antibiotics and get better in one week, versus seven days without antibiotics." We need to save antibiotics for life-saving infectious situations.

Last but not least is the fact that all pharmaceuticals are tested on animals. Mahatma Gandhi said, "The greatness of a society and its moral progress can be judged by the way it treats its animals." Our society should be embarrassed.

Millions of animals are sacrificed every year to study new drugs. The animals are kept in deplorable conditions, are under constant stress, and are literally tortured, all for the purpose of testing the newest blood pressure drug or chemotherapy agent. Defenders of this practice will point to all the lives saved from animal cruelty. This excuse is just a clever marketing trick, as drugs and surgery barely increased our lifespan. Sanitation, clear water, and quality food are the reasons we live until 80. The money, time, people, and other resources used on animal research should be allocated to health education and prevention. Think about these living creatures, all feeling pain and suffering, the next time you reach for a Tylenol or Advil.

Given what we just discussed, what is the evidence drugs used in cardiology lead to any benefit? We heard from the drug companies for years with their constant advertising and we heard from our doctors who practice mindless pharmaceutical medicine. Now follow me as we look at the current state of heart care.

DRUGS TO REDUCE CHOLESTEROL

Cholesterol is the waxy, life-giving molecule mainly produced in the liver. We described its benefits in Chapter 1. A chain of reactions occurs to form cholesterol, with the enzyme HMG CoA reductase a major link in the chain. A class of drugs known to inhibit this enzyme are affectionately known as statins, based on the fact the generic names of these drugs contain the suffix "statin." Millions of people take statins to lower cholesterol and presumably lower cardiac risk. Billions of dollars were collected from the sales of Lipitor, Crestor, Zocor, etc. Yet is there any proof of their benefit?

The fact statins lower cholesterol and LDL is not up for debate. They do, and sometimes dramatically so. Unfortunately for our brain, our hormones, our digestive tract, and every cell in our body, statins decrease the pool of cholesterol available. There is little information regarding the long-term effects of this class of drugs. We do know the extensive list of side effects includes diabetes, cataracts, muscle damage, liver damage, and low testosterone, to name just a few. Those on statins should be monitored for liver and kidney damage every three months.

Let's take a closer look at statins to decipher the benefits of this class of drug. One of the first large studies to assess this question was AFCAPS/TEXCAPS.[99] This study, released in 1998, was a primary prevention trial with over six thousand participants without any known heart disease. Half the group received the statin drug Pravastatin and the other half a placebo (not active treatment). The results changed medicine as we know it, so brace yourself for these results (you might want to sit or lay down with this book!). The earth-shattering difference between groups regarding cardiac events was 4.9% in the drug group versus 6.4% in the placebo group. This was a grand total of 1.5% difference after 5 years on the drug.

I am not impressed with 1.5%. Another way to look at this data is 63 people need to take the drug for 5 years in order to prevent 1 person from having an event. This important and illuminating statistic is called a "number needed to treat," or NNT. Always ask for this information from your doctor regarding any therapy. One last amazing statistic for this group of patients—if 63 people take the drug for 5 years, 114,975 pills would be consumed to prevent 1 event! That is a lot of pills, and a lot of money for Big Pharma.

But get this folks, the most important finding from AFCAPS was the number of people who died was the SAME in each group! Statins did not prevent deaths from overall causes. In the statin group, fewer people died of heart disease, yet more were likely to die from cancer and suicide. This critical information was glossed over by cardiologists, causing the spigots of statin production to open like floodgates. I guess cardiologists aren't concerned how you die, as long as it is not heart related.

You might like to know that AFCAPS was funded by Merck, the manufacturer of Pravastatin. Is it possible the people who fund a study can tamper with the results? This question should be asked about every study. We need to look beyond the headlines and see the motivation of the authors. Do you think it is possible a corporate executive could alter data in favor of the drug group? What do you think happens to the researcher who brings negative results to the corporate CEO when billions of dollars are on the line?

★**LIVE WELL**: AFCAPS was funded by Merck, the manufacturer of Pravastatin. No lives were saved by taking the drug.

Why don't doctors realize this snow job? There are many factors involved but in general, doctors are so busy seeing patients every ten minutes there is no time to read, and if they do, it is an article in a journal sponsored by pharmaceutical companies. The drug reps come in the office, stuff our faces, and show beautiful charts touting the glories of their pills. Medical doctors are no match for the powerful marketing efforts of corporations. They know our patterns and behaviors better than we know ourselves. I was very close with Big Pharma reps who revealed to me the detailed training involved in coercion. The reps are like highly skilled ninjas.

In 1995, the results of the West of Scotland trial were released. This study looked at over 6,000 men over a period of five years whose average total cholesterol was over 270. Half the group received Pravastatin 40mg and half got the placebo. The findings from this study, along with AFCAPS, would propel American doctors to strong-arm their patients into the use of statin drugs. Unfortunately, women also received this recommendation, although scarce data exists to imply a benefit in females.

West of Scotland showed after five years, the statin group had a 3.2% chance of dying versus a 4.1% chance. The number needed to treat (NNT) was 110 for this end-point, which again means that 110 people must take the drug for five years to prevent one death. According to my calculations, over 200,000 Pravastatin capsules must be swallowed over five years to prevent one death. Heart attacks decreased from 7.8% to 5.8%.[100] The drug worked, but not by much. Again, I am not here to argue whether or not statins lower risk; the data suggests they do (unless you think corporate America would "doctor" the results for obvious reasons). My mission is to suggest to patients there is a way to reduce events much further with a goal of 0% event rates.

In 2008 the results of the JUPITER trial were released. This study examined patients with an elevated CRP (a marker of inflammation) and thus an increased cardiovascular risk. Half the group received the cholesterol drug rosuvastatin and the other half a placebo. The drug group had a lower chance of dying, 2.2% vs. 2.8% after two years.[101] This trivial difference was dwarfed by news media sensationalism claiming thousands of lives would be saved if people took this drug.

★**LIVE WELL**: Over 200,000 Pravastatin capsules must be swallowed over five years to prevent one death.

Admittedly, the statin data gets a little better using drugs for secondary prevention, where trial participants have a history of a heart attack, angioplasty, or bypass surgery. Merck sponsored the 4S trial, which demonstrated a reduction in events from 22.6% to 15.9%. This led to a NNT of 16, where 16 people take the drug for over 5 years to prevent one event. The risk of death was reduced by 4%.[102] These numbers are not insignificant. Statin trials, especially in secondary prevention, show benefit. I am not here to argue this point (although conspiracy theorists may claim drug makers control the data). What I am here to say and what my medical practice is based upon is that there is a BETTER way to prevent and treat heart disease without potentially dangerous pharmaceuticals. The goal is not to reduce risk from 22% to 16%. The goal is to reduce risk to 0%. Despite drugs, 10% of patients died within five years of enrollment. Doctors must offer a better solution. Patients need to demand a change. Heart disease does not occur because the body lacks Lipitor, Crestor, or Zocor. All disease is from poor nutrition and chemicals, sprinkled with stress and inactivity.

Now for the downside of drugs. I consulted on many patients who are intolerant of statins or suffered their side effects. Some, like my patient Tom for example, had severe muscle damage from a statin drug. Even years after stopping the offending medication, Tom still has weakness and pain in his muscles. Thousands of patients developed severe muscle and liver damage from statin drugs. Other patients complain of memory loss and transient amnesia. These people literally lose all recollection for days at a time! An excellent book was written several years ago by Duane Graveline M.D. titled *Lipitor: Thief of Memory*. In his book, Dr. Graveline documents dozens of patients with memory issues from statin drugs. I personally think these people fall through the cracks (are covered up) in large trials ALL paid for by Big Pharma.

Once again, the issue at hand is that statins limit the production of cholesterol, a critical molecule for cell function, hormone formation, digestion, and vitamin D production. There is no wonder why memory loss and amnesia occur in people on these drugs. Every cell in the body is dependent on cholesterol. Human life is not possible without cholesterol, even though it gets such a bad rap. Statins and other drugs for cholesterol do not address the cause of disease, thus representing another Band-Aid approach.

★LIVE WELL: The goal in treating heart disease is to find the CAUSE and reduce risk to 0%.

DRUGS TO REDUCE BLOOD PRESSURE

"Your blood pressure is so high you're going to have a stroke!" Medical doctors are great at scare tactics geared toward getting patients on drugs to lower blood pressure. Big Pharma shows an ad with a guy drooling in his wheelchair to hammer home the point. I am not saying high blood pressure is a good thing and hypertension certainly is not normal, nor is it the sign of a healthy person. Elevated blood pressure (BP) is a sign of disease, not a disease itself. The cause is not a beta-blocker or ACE inhibitor deficiency. Poor nutrition and chemicals are the causes, along with lack of physical activity, poor sleep, and increased stress.

Elevated blood pressure or hypertension puts a person at increased risk over their lifetime for heart attacks, stroke, kidney failure, and death. The increased risk is seen in people with elevated blood pressure for many years. This fact, however, allows patients time to change their lifestyle and use supplements to achieve a better blood pressure reading. Hypertension is a sign of endothelial dysfunction (ED, not erectile dysfunction, which actually has the same cause). When these endothelial cells lining the blood vessel are not functioning normally, it can result in elevated blood pressure. Again, patients can improve endothelial function with nutrition and supplements.

Sadly, the majority of doctors will not heed my advice. Instead, they will quickly pull out their prescription pad to write for the drug whose drug rep recently bought them lunch. Why spend time discussing prevention tactics such as dramatic blood pressure reductions through nutrition and exercise? Beets, nuts, carb restriction, omega 3 fats, and dozens of other foods lower blood pressure. Additionally, chiropractic care, acupuncture, meditation, and yoga are proven to lower blood pressure.

★**LIVE WELL**: There are many ways to lower blood pressure naturally.

So if your blood pressure is high, should you go on drugs? Most doctors will urge this course of action (which we were all trained to do), but what is the benefit? I will explain some data to you, but it is interesting that in early 2014, the blood pressure guidelines were revised. The blood pressure at which drugs are recommended was moved to above 150 systolic (the top number) and 90 diastolic (bottom number).[103] This means millions of men and women no longer need to take pills with all the risk and minimal benefit. How much money has Big Pharma stuffed in their pockets on the backs of those patients who never really needed the drug? Drugs can dramatically lower blood pressure, but do they decrease your chance of heart attacks, stroke, or dying? This is the question we need to ask. Why was your blood pressure medication started?

Most trials conclude blood pressure drugs do not lower heart attack risk. A 2014 trial found no reduction in heart attacks amongst patients on antihypertensive drugs.[104] So if the drugs do not decrease heart attack risk, why take them? Well, maybe they reduce strokes. Stroke was also an endpoint in the above trial, and the drugs did work. Stroke risk decreased from 5.5% to 5%. Number needed to treat, 200. Not very impressive.

★**LIVE WELL**: New guidelines suggest millions of men and women no longer need pills for high blood pressure.

The SYST EUR trial examined pharmaceuticals vs. placebo in patients with an average blood pressure of 173 systolic. After several years, 94.9% of the drug group were alive versus 94.1% of the placebo group.[105] This subtle difference should not cause us to drive to the pharmacy, but rather to walk the aisles of a healthy grocer. Another trial, using the drug candesartan (Atacand), actually found an increased rate of cancer and heart attacks in the pharma group.[106] This drug is still widely used over a decade after this trial was published. In fact, a recent review found the entire class of drugs similar to candesartan were linked to a higher cancer risk.[107] Read the last sentence again: CANCER.

The HOPE trial looked at high-risk patients with diabetes or vascular disease and gave them an ACE inhibitor or placebo.[108] After five years, more people were alive in the drug group, but only by 1.8%, with a NNT of 56. Again, this means 56 people must take drug for 5 years in order for one event to be prevented. 55 people will take the drug and receive no benefit at all, yet be exposed to countless side effects. Even in this group of people at the highest risk, benefits were minimal. The stock of King Pharmaceuticals soared when the trial results were released.

One 2014 study revealed that a person who takes blood pressure medication has a 40% increased risk of falling. Of those who had a serious injury after a fall, 17% died! How sad millions of elderly people are overmedicated for minimal benefit, and yet must endure all the risk.[109] Another recent study showed when pharmaceuticals markedly lower blood pressure, the risk of cancer dramatically increased by 260%. The cause of this association is yet to be determined, but I would play it safe and avoid drugs. Why risk your health by waiting to find the cause?[110]

Are you getting the picture? Drugs to lower your blood pressure provide minimal benefit, yet may result in profound risks to your overall health. Several drugs in this class were banned by the FDA (years after approval) or relegated to obscurity because of intolerable side effects. One banned drug was Posicor, found to increase deaths after some time on the market. Check out the side effects of drugs like reserpine, methyldopa, and hydralazine. In fact, check out the side effects of all drugs. Read about them on your own, not in the blazing 10 seconds at the end of a commercial.

★**LIVE WELL**: Drugs to lower blood pressure may cause serious harm.

ASPIRIN

There are many examples of commonly used pharmaceuticals with trivial to zero benefit. Aspirin is one of those drugs, swallowed by tens of millions of people for the supposed prevention of heart attack and stroke. It is the single biggest sham drug in history. The American College of Cardiology specifically recommends aspirin not be used in healthy women under 65. The drug has small benefits for those who already suffered a heart attack. Why ingest a drug with minimal benefit that poses a substantial bleeding risk? At least 15 people DIE of a gastrointestinal bleed for every 100,000 who take aspirin.[111] Let's find out more.

An interesting study found aspirin given to a healthy 74-year-old man would reduce his annual risk of a cardiovascular event from 2% to 1.74% (absolute risk reduction is 0.26%, number needed to treat is 385). That means over 140,000 aspirins must be choked down to prevent one event. That same man taking aspirin would increase his gastrointestinal bleeding risk from 0.3% to 0.51% (absolute risk increase is 0.21%, number needed to harm is 4/6).[112] Do you believe this lunacy? The heart doctors are happy with miniscule benefits, while the GI doctors are thrilled with the increased business from the bleeders. The Bayer Corporation has the audacity to claim it prevents 1 out of 3 heart attacks! The commercials are all over television. Where is the FDA, and why aren't they going after this false advertising? I can't claim a multivitamin is beneficial because of the FDA, but Bayer can get away with lies and blatantly misleading information.

On May 5, 2014, the FDA banned Bayer from recommending aspirin for the primary prevention of a heart attack or stroke. The FDA did not find evidence supporting aspirin use for those who never had a heart attack or stroke. This earth shattering statement, and clear rebuff of the Bayer Corporation, affects millions of people currently taking this drug. That's right, aspirin is a drug. Sadly, millions of people take this dangerous drug for muscle and joint pain when there are many natural options. What is more important is finding the cause of pain (gluten and other food sensitivities for example).

In addition to GI bleeding here are a few other side effects of aspirin:

1. Increases uric acid, which can lead to gout, a painful form of arthritis. When people are in pain, they swallow more aspirin.[113]
2. Decreases kidney function.[114]
3. Leads to blindness. Aspirin increases the risk of the "wet" form of macular degeneration, which is a leading cause of blindness in older people.[115]
4. Increases the risk of blood clots in surgical patients.[116]
5. Leads to hearing loss.[117]

★ **LIVE WELL**: The side effects of aspirin use for heart disease are far greater than the benefits, especially for women.

OTHER BLOOD THINNERS

If you are unfortunate enough to wind up with a scrap of metal called a stent in your heart artery, a drug similar to aspirin is added. The most common of this class is clopidogrel, which has a trade name of Plavix. This drug has very modest benefit of keeping stents open when added to aspirin alone for the first year. Only a 3% reduction of events was noted in studies involving the Plavix/aspirin group versus aspirin alone. After one year, little data supports any benefit to continuing on this aggressive blood thinner. Yet, the typical cardiologist tells patients to remain on this drug after the one-year mark, citing little downside. Sure, the only downside is double the bleeding risk when combined with aspirin versus aspirin alone. In fact, a recent study found those who continued on this class of drugs, which includes Effient and Brillinta, for more than a year had a higher risk of death.[118] I stop this drug between 6-12 months after a stent in every patient.

Medical bills are often cited as the number one cause of bankruptcy. Plavix, even generic, can cost a fortune. It is also known to interfere with other drugs, therefore increasing the danger of horrific bleeding. Some people are genetically predisposed to an increased bleeding risk on many drugs. There are genetic tests to guide the safety of blood thinners, but doctors rarely take the time to discover this information. Prior to Plavix was a drug named Ticlid, which the FDA finally pulled after several patients died.

★**LIVE WELL**: Plavix is effective in keeping stents open for the first year only.

Another nasty player in the blood thinning toolbox is warfarin. Commonly known as Coumadin, this drug is used for stroke prevention in patients with atrial fibrillation. This drug started its career as rat poison (no joke). Coumadin is extremely overprescribed and only benefits those with the highest stroke risk. Stroke risk for the majority of people on the drug is reduced from 4% to 2.5%. Bleeding on warfarin can be catastrophic and deadly. It has significant food interactions and therefore must be monitored closely. Antibiotics, for example, can markedly affect drug levels and lead to a subsequent loss of blood. I saw this many times as a hospital physician over the years. New drugs on the market, such as Pradaxa and Xarelto, thin the blood, but there is no antidote that can reverse their blood-thinning effects in the case of an emergency bleed. The ambulance chasing attorneys are all over this drug class. Why take a drug with minimal benefit and so much risk? I love getting my patients off these dangerous pharmaceuticals. Please ask your doctor if this approach is correct for you.

DRUGS FOR HEART RHYTHM

A common complaint in the cardiologist's office is palpitations. Patients describe feelings of their heart racing, skipping, or thumping. Although there are many causes, these symptoms are often due to extra heartbeats called PVC's, or premature ventricular complexes. Our friends at Big Pharma have an answer to everything, and for years a class of drugs known as anti-arrhythmics were used. In 1992, a study was published looking at patients with a previous heart attack and suppressing their PVC's. This landmark trial, known as CAST, found those taking the active drug died at three times the rate as a placebo.[119] How many died from the use of this class of drugs is unknown, but given they were available for many years, the number is likely in the thousands. Though this trial was more than 20 years ago, the point remains valid: who is watching out for the consumer? Others drugs require the patient to be hospitalized for days to monitor for safety.

The sad situation regarding dangerous drugs is natural supplements, such as magnesium, potassium, omega 3 oils, and other nutrients, can remedy the situation. Once again, it is about finding the cause. Extra heartbeats can arise from nutrient deficiencies and metals/toxins, but are never the result of a lack of pharmaceuticals. I treat patients whose symptoms resolved after eliminating caffeine, gluten, or corn. For others, it may be a sign of sensitivity to dairy or eggs. Patients must demand their doctor find the CAUSE. I am successful because I find the cause.

> ★LIVE WELL: Your morning coffee or afternoon sugar snack could be the cause of your symptoms.

DIABETES DRUGS

Let us talk briefly about Type 2 diabetes. Over 20 million Americans carry this diagnosis of elevated blood sugar, which increases the risk of heart disease, strokes, cancer, and dementia. Elevated blood sugar is from eating sugar and carbs! Combine poor nutrition with chemicals and: 1) the pancreas cannot produce enough insulin, 2) the tissues of the body become resistant to insulin. Insulin is the key that opens the door to cells allowing energy (as glucose, protein, and fat) to enter. When blood sugar is too high for too long, insulin becomes the key that can no longer fit in the lock and open the door.

Corporations know people don't want to change their diet or exercise, so pharmaceuticals are developed to lower blood sugar. Tens of billions are spent on this class of drug every year to keep levels under control. But as we saw with statins and blood pressure pills, lowering numbers does not necessarily lower cardiac events. A trial called ACCORD looked at this very issue of intensive blood sugar control in patients with type 2 diabetes. The authors found a 22% increased risk of death in the group with the best blood sugar control![120] Those same investigators also found blood pressure reduction in diabetics with a goal below 120mmHg did not provide any additional benefit than those who achieved a blood pressure below 140mmHg.[121] Sometimes, getting too aggressive does not pay off in health dividends.

Questions remain as to why this therapy increased mortality, but it is reassuring to those with diabetes that the answer is actually quite simple—stop eating sugar and carbohydrates, which cause diabetes and high blood pressure in the first place! Eat Paleo and watch your blood sugar normalize and cardiac risk go down. I witnessed this in my patients thousands of times, and it can happen for you as well.

Take my patient Ray M. for example. His fasting blood sugar at our first visit was 145. After three months on Paleo nutrition, his blood sugar was 96. It is so simple.

★**LIVE WELL**: Drugs designed for reducing diabetes and high blood pressure do not necessarily lower the risk of cardiac events.

A HISTORY OF FAILED DRUGS

How many dozens of drugs has the FDA approved only to be subsequently recalled and banned? How many people died from:

- Hismanal—for allergies
- Baycol—for cholesterol
- Propulsid—for reflux/heartburn
- Posicor—for hypertension
- Avandia—for diabetes
- Trovafloxacin—for infections
- Thalidomide—for morning sickness

This list is literally hundreds of drugs long. During my residency, we passed out Trovafloxacin and Baycol as if they were candy. Anyone who was even slightly overweight was offered a prescription for Fen-Phen, until the drug was pulled by the FDA (it was cited for increased cardiovascular risks). The maker of the Fen part of the combo had legal ramifications to the tune of almost 4 billion dollars![122]

How many millions suffered the dreaded side effects of pharmaceuticals that were CORRECTLY prescribed? In 1994, a study found over 100,000 people died from correctly prescribed drugs.[123] Actually, drugs don't cause side effects. They are chemicals that do not know what they are supposed to do. They just go into the body and "effect" things. How many thousands needlessly die from incorrectly prescribed drugs and pharmacy errors? The pill-for–every-ill mentality must stop. The human body is the best pharmacy, as it knows exactly what to produce at exactly the right time. Just put in the correct fuel.

While I am on a roll, the benefit of drugs used for dementia, arthritis, and even cancer amount to trivial benefit, if any at all. For example, Tamiflu, a drug to fight the flu, was shown (in a study paid for by the manufacturer) to reduce flu symptoms from 7 to 6 days. Yes, you read this correctly. Tamiflu cut the duration by 1 day. If you watch TV, advertisers seem to claim this sham of a product prevents everything from the common cold to HIV. The government has amassed billions of dollars' worth of this drug in case of a national emergency. Do you think the manufacturer has the ear of the politician in charge of ordering this drug? They have that ear because of campaign contributions and other perks.

Two eye-opening books that influenced my transformation to a natural doctor were *Overdosed* by John Abramson, MD, and *The Truth about Drug Companies* by Marcia Angell, MD. The latter was the first woman editor-in-chief of the prestigious *New England Journal of Medicine*, who then turned whistleblower. There are more of us speaking out than ever before, and surely others will follow to topple the sickness paradigm ironically referred to as the American health system.

Medical doctors and pharmaceutical companies keep promising the mythical polypill to prevent disease. This magic combination of different drugs in a single capsule will allow us to eat all the crap we want while we sit on our toxic couch, smoking cigars, and drinking beer or wine. The public waits with bated breath. But when will the synthetic health elixir be available? The answer is never. Only prevention with nutrition, chemical avoidance, detoxification, de-stress, and exercise will truly make a difference. There are no shortcuts.

Take my patient Sheila who, at the age of 47, was on several drugs. She came to see me when she heard I look for the cause of disease and get people off pharmaceuticals. She felt fatigued and had muscle soreness since starting on her drugs over two years ago. She believed her memory was not as sharp, and she had trouble with name recall and finding her car keys. Also, heartburn plagued her for the last few months.

The first pill I immediately stopped was Fosamax, a drug used in patients with osteoporosis for fracture prevention. I explained to Sheila osteoporosis was not a disease of Fosamax deficiency, it was from poor nutrition, lack of exercise, and chemicals. We stopped it immediately because the benefit of the drug is trivial at best and fraught with side effects, including the heartburn she experienced. She was also on a pill for cholesterol and a pill for high blood pressure. Sheila provided me with a history of never having a blood pressure above 150 systolic, yet her previous doctor felt drugs were necessary. The same doctor prescribed a statin drug because her total cholesterol was over 200; "My wife takes it" was his final push for Sheila. We stopped both pills immediately. The only pharmaceutical that remained was thyroid, which we would successfully stop in the near future.

After eliminating the above-mentioned drugs, within one month Sheila was a new woman. Today, with nutrition, supplements, exercise, and chemical avoidance, her "numbers" are normal. In fact, she is taking courses to become a health coach to teach others about alternatives to conventional medicine's pills and procedures.

Martha P. came to see me for hypertension and wanted to get off her two pharmaceuticals. With dietary changes, adding beetroot powder, taurine, and magnesium, stress reduction, and improved sleep duration, the drugs were able to be stopped. You read correctly, beetroot powder. How easy is that? However, I am not trying to convince you to go at it alone. Natural remedies can be very powerful and can lead to some unpleasant side effects. Seek consultation from a natural doctor who has the experience of thousands of patients to call upon. Each person is unique, and in-depth knowledge is required to get you on the correct health path.

ACTION PLAN

Here is a quick checklist of questions for your doctor when prescribing pharmaceuticals for any condition:

1. What are we doing to address the cause of my condition?
2. Are there any natural alternatives to the drug you are recommending?
3. What are the studies showing this drug is effective?
4. What is the number needed to treat (NNT)? My favorite.
5. What are the side effects?
6. How will you monitor the side effects?

You, as the consumer and the patient, must ask your doctor serious questions and demand answers. Your doctor will not like to be questioned since they are not accustomed to any interrogation, and frankly don't have the time during your 10-minute visit. Frequently, the doctor does not know the answer. If these are issues with your current healthcare provider, you need to find one who can work with you as part of a team with the goal of a long, happy, healthy, and drug-free life.

Chapter 7

USELESS DANGEROUS PROCEDURES

"Never go to a doctor whose office plants have died."
—Erma Bombeck

S how up at any radiology-testing center and the line will be out the door. Women anxiously line up for mammograms, while routine chest x-rays are performed along with countless CT scans and MRI's. The reality is that these tests are dangerous and usually unnecessary, but always financially rewarding to the doctor. Let's look at the example of mammograms. A 2014 study from the most prestigious medical journal in the world, *JAMA*, found one life will be saved if 1,000 women each get a mammogram yearly for 10 years.[124] Screening leads to false-positives where the result is abnormal, but the patient does not have cancer. Yet, the patient is subjected to additional procedures and biopsies, causing tremendous stress and anxiety. Yes, you may be the 1 out of

1,000. Or, you could be one of the hundreds exposed to dangerous follow-up testing. Breast cancer is an emotionally charged subject. Contrary to popular belief, the actual causes are poor nutrition and excessive use of chemicals. The radiologists, who make a fortune off female scare tactics, are very protective of their turf.

A large part of my cardiology training was learning how to perform and interpret cardiovascular tests. Treadmills, echocardiograms, nuclear imaging, angiography etc. were very exciting procedures for the aspiring cardiologist. After I joined a large cardiology group, however, I soon learned the real importance of these procedures—they make money … lots of money. Let's take a closer look at the risks and benefits of heart testing.

★**LIVE WELL**: Mammograms barely save lives and lead to tremendous stress and anxiety.

STRESS TESTING

Stress testing is an excellent way to determine if a person's symptoms are heart related. The noninvasive treadmill provides information about exercise capacity, blood pressure, and heart rate. If someone develops chest pain or shortness of breath at a low workload, a blockage may be likely and further testing could be necessary. After years on the couch, a treadmill stress test is useful prior to starting an exercise routine. One particularly weak indication for a stress test is prior to surgery. Pre-operative stress tests are usually worthless, often delaying surgery (which could be a good thing). If the stress test is abnormal, an angiogram could lead to a stent, which leads to a blood thinner, which means you can't go through surgery. This scenario may sound reasonable, but if you dig deeper, you will learn stents do not prevent heart attacks (more on this issue in the next couple of pages).

★**LIVE WELL**: Stress testing is a huge money-maker for cardiologists and hospitals.

The problem is that for years cardiologists milked the system. These tests are ordered needlessly just to line the pockets of the doc. For some reason, insurance companies paid cardiologists outrageous sums of money for performing this test. A plain treadmill test does not pay well, but a treadmill test with nuclear imaging? That was money in the bank. I was highly "encouraged" to order this test for years. Recently, insurance companies and Medicare are denying routine stress testing, recognizing it is unnecessary.

Nuclear imaging involves radioactive material injected directly into the body. This test is commonly known as a thallium stress test. The nuclear exam is often falsely positive, meaning everything is actually fine but the test was incorrectly abnormal. This usually leads to a dangerous and unnecessary angiogram. Nuclear imaging adds very little in the majority of cases, but certainly adds expense and plenty of radiation. If your doctor pushes an imaging technique, opt for a stress echocardiogram. This ultrasound of your heart provides more information without the radiation.

★**LIVE WELL**: Bottom line: if your baseline ECG is normal and you can perform on a treadmill, nuclear imaging is not necessary.

In a recent study published in the *Journal of the American Medical Association* involving patients taken to the ER with chest pain, those hospitals that performed the most nuclear scans had the same outcomes (patients with heart attacks or who died) as those who did the least amount of scans. Hospitals that perform the most stress tests also do an enormous amount of angiograms and stents. But once again, this behavior does not prevent any heart attacks or save lives.[125] I want to stress this again: if you have symptoms, the only test you need is a treadmill stress test, provided you can perform on a treadmill and your baseline ECG is relatively normal. When pushed into a procedure, ask for a second opinion if you are uncomfortable.

★**LIVE WELL**: When considering most heart procedures, always seek a second opinion.

CT SCANS

One test called the EBCT, or coronary calcium scan, became very popular in the late '90s. This test involves x-rays to determine the amount of calcification in the coronary arteries. The more calcium present, the more coronary artery disease. Calcium is left as a remnant of inflammation and cellular death. The scan is noninvasive, which makes it more attractive than the invasive coronary angiography. Your coronary calcium score is used to determine your risk of cardiovascular events such as heart attacks, strokes, and death. More calcium leads to a higher score and therefore a higher risk.

Many trials looked at the added value of CT scans. Do they help identify risk in individuals over and above other risk factors such as age, weight, sex, lipids, diabetes, smoking, inflammation, family history, etc.? In my opinion, based on the data, the answer is no. Even if the CT scan does identify people with and without coronary disease, my treatment strategy is the same. I assume everyone has coronary disease because the vast majority of people do. I find the fact that insurance companies typically do not pay for this test indicative of its lack of a clear benefit. Peddlers of this form of radiation scan dropped the price considerably, in some cases to $99 or less.

For example, will a high or low calcium score change the therapy of the average cardiologist? The answer is no. Statin drugs are the only treatment doctors recommend, and they are unlikely to be influenced by the CT scan score. A 2014 study found those patients with a high calcium score, but no other risk factors, did NOT benefit from statin drugs.[126] Your doctor should be advocating aggressive lifestyle changes, such as Paleo nutrition, physical activity, and relaxation.

★**LIVE WELL**: Coronary CT scans expose the patient to high levels of radiation and do not provide enough information to warrant the risk.

An unfortunate consequence of the calcium CT scan is that it leads to further unnecessary tests such as stress testing and angiography. A patient could wind up with coronary stents or even bypass surgery when no symptoms were ever experienced. A common misconception is that opening up blocked vessels prevents heart attacks, or keeps people from dying. It doesn't. In fact, stents may increase the risk. Check out the COURAGE trial published in the *New England Journal of Medicine* in 2007. Stents are for symptoms and do not prevent heart attacks or save lives. Why do cardiologists still stent everything in sight? Follow the money: Stress testing, angiography, stents, and bypass surgery are very lucrative.

★**LIVE WELL**: Unless you are in the midst of a heart attack, a stent will not save your life. Stents are for symptoms, but there is a better way.

Lastly, the CT scan is a source of significant radiation, equivalent to around 200-400 chest x-rays. Sure, doctors will deny radiation dangers (personally I would not want one chest x-ray), but it is clear the more CT scans in your life, the higher your cancer risk. Radiation damages all tissues, which is the reason medical personnel take extreme precautions to limit radiation exposure. Researchers at the National Cancer Institute estimate 29,000 future cancer cases could be attributed to the 72 million CT scans performed in the country in 2007.[127] A 2009 study of medical centers in the San Francisco Bay Area also calculated an elevated risk: one extra case of cancer for every 400 to 2,000 routine chest CT exams. Radiation causes damage to DNA, destroys the integrity of blood vessels, and is a likely cause of coronary disease.

Since most adults harbor some degree of coronary artery disease, why get the CT scan? Just assume you have some level of disease and move forward with trying to prevent any further progression. The best way to good health is through eating nutritious foods and avoiding chemicals. Take high quality supplements and get the toxins out of your body. Go for advanced blood analysis to uncover risk markers that are modifiable with nutrition and supplements. And, of course, don't forget to exercise and de-stress.

If you do get radiated by CT or nuclear injection, take an anti-oxidant supplement before and after the procedure. There is plenty of evidence these supplements prevent radiation damage.

★**LIVE WELL**: Radiation destroys the integrity of your blood vessels and can cause coronary disease.

ANGIOGRAMS

Angiogram, or heart catheterization, is an invasive procedure where tubes are inserted into arteries to determine if a blockage is present. As you can imagine, this is a very risky test with the possibility of the doctor causing a heart attack, stroke, or death. I witnessed those complications many times in my career. Injury to the femoral artery at the insertion site can lead to long-term numbness and pain. Unfortunately, in one case years ago, I tried to save a woman who died from bleeding at the angiogram puncture site. This is a very dangerous test. Angiography also exposes the patient to a massive amount of radiation. Many patients leave the catheterization lab with burn marks on their backs. Radiation causes cancer. Sure, you sign a consent form, which includes these risks, but does anyone actually explain them to you?

When you are in the midst of a heart attack, an angiogram is a great test, for it offers therapy in the form of angioplasty and a stent. A heart attack is the only situation where stents save lives (an exception may be stenting the Left Main as I will discuss in a few paragraphs). Unfortunately, heart catheterizations are needlessly performed thousands of times per year on patients who never had a symptom in their life. The only indication for the angiogram was an abnormal stress test, itself a likely unnecessary test. Recently, the journal *Circulation: Interventions* reported data from New York that concluded 25% of angiograms were inappropriate. Another whopping 40% were of "uncertain appropriateness"![128] Get this reader: doctors earn money by doing tests and procedures. This behavior has led to some very rich physicians. When in doubt, ask for a second opinion, or a third opinion.

In my practice, I offer patients an alternative. Let's say a patient has chest discomfort with exertion. The typical cardiologist will send for an angiogram.

But what if we can treat with nutrition and supplements to minimize symptoms? Most patients gain a significant relief of chest pain and improvement in shortness of breath with simple lifestyle changes such as good nutrition, supplements, and chemical avoidance. Patients of mine get chest pain relief from L-arginine, beetroot powder, and hawthorn. Seek out a doctor who can offer a natural approach without the use of dangerous procedures. Consult with a holistic practitioner, and then decide on the best plan.

★LIVE WELL: Angiograms are often unnecessary and carry health risks including radiation exposure, stroke, kidney failure, and death. Nutrition and supplements are a better solution.

STENTS

The only indication for a stent is in a patient with symptoms. In my experience, nutrition and supplements can be very useful in patients with chest pain and shortness of breath, making a stent unnecessary. It can be very difficult, however, for a patient to comprehend that a severe blockage is not going to lead to a heart attack. But the fact is, the more the artery is blocked, the less likely it is to cause heart damage because the blockage is STABLE. It may cause symptoms, but not a heart attack. The heart attack comes from when a mild blockage suddenly ruptures, leading to loss of blood flow to part of the heart.

Do all patients with chest pain need a stent? This was the question posed in the COURAGE trial published in 2007 in the *New England Journal of Medicine*.[129] The study divided a group of patients with cardiac symptoms into two groups: one included stenting and pharmaceuticals, and the other with only pharmaceuticals. The results revealed stenting did not prevent heart attacks or death. In fact, the stent group had slightly more heart attacks. Medical therapy was just as good as stents without all the risk. Do you think this changed the behavior of any cardiologists? Not one bit. Rarely does the interventional cardiologist pass up the opportunity to put metal in the arteries. Once again, this is putting cash right into the doctor's pocket, and insurance companies pay for it without question. It is just the cost of doing business to them, as they pass on the cost to those of us who pay insurance.

Unnecessary procedures for Medicare and Medicaid patients are billed to the American taxpayer.

★**LIVE WELL**: Stents do not prevent heart attacks, but they CAN cause them.

Be careful because hospital doctors love to scare people into procedures that may not be necessary. The patient is put into a very difficult situation. In most cases, there is still time to make a decision and seek a consultation with a natural doctor, or at least the opinion of a doctor in a different group. The question we need to ask is, can nutrition and supplements outperform pharmaceuticals and stents? I firmly believe the answer is yes. Natural doctors have been doing this for years. If you remove and avoid toxins while feeding your body the correct fuel, you will heal.

★**LIVE WELL**: Take away the cause of the problem and the body will heal itself.

BYPASS SURGERY

Coronary artery bypass graft (CABG) surgery is the granddaddy of them all. This abused procedure takes place hundreds of thousands of times per year, usually unnecessarily. We have known for many years that open-heart surgery should only be done in a select few cases, but this surgery pays a fortune. In the '80s and '90s, heart surgeons were making millions of dollars per year. The gravy train was running full tilt. Surgeons were the "heroes" to millions of Americans whose lives were supposedly saved. This was actually far from the truth.

The study, which should have put a halt to this abuse, was the CASS trial.[130] The researchers took a group of patients with cardiac symptoms along with significant heart disease and divided them into two groups: those who had surgery and those without surgery. In this breakthrough study, the only individuals with improved life expectancy from surgery were those with Left Main disease or multi-vessel disease with left ventricular dysfunction(heart doesn't pump well).

The Left Main is the artery supplying most of the heart. A blockage there is not something to trivialize. Fortunately, it is not very common, and represents a small portion of bypass patients.

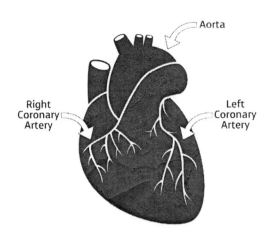

People with one or two vessel disease (there are three major vessels) with normal heart function do not live any longer with surgery than without it. Would these same people fare better with drastic nutrition, lifestyle, and supplement intervention? Definitely, but don't hold your breath for the study. Contrary to the above mentioned CASS trial, another trial in 2011 found minimal benefit after six years in those with severe coronary disease AND left ventricular dysfunction. In fact, after the first two years, the death rate was higher in the surgical group! Don't take my word for it, look up the article and bring it to your doctor.[131] Here's my advice—consider surgery or a stent for severe left main coronary artery disease. Otherwise, seek out the help of a natural doctor to avoid surgery.

★LIVE WELL: Open-heart surgery is beneficial to only a small portion of its recipients. If you had open heart bypass, you probably did not need it.

Do you think the results of the CASS trial changed patterns of practice? Hardly, and I know this because I witnessed these surgeries on a daily basis. When cardiologists see blockage, their response is always stents or surgery. The landmark CASS trial demonstrated, in patients with three vessels blocked and normal heart function (ejection fraction), a heart bypass did not improve their life expectancy. Yet these people are the ones so commonly sent to bypass surgery. You see, the surgeons and the cardiologists are all good friends, enjoying lavish parties funded on the cracked chests of unassuming patients. Sorry to those of you with "zippers" where your sternum should be, but these are the facts.

Bypass surgery is a procedure with well-documented complications, including but not limited to:

1. Death
2. Stroke
3. Heart attack
4. Kidney failure
5. Memory loss
6. Chronic chest pain
7. Lung damage
8. Vocal cord damage

Sometimes surgery is needed. There is no other treatment for very tight heart valves or very leaky heart valves. Patients with large aneurysms should undergo surgical repair. But patients need to understand the risks and benefits of any procedure.

★LIVE WELL: The risks associated with open-heart surgery usually outweigh the benefits.

ABLATION

There are a few different types of abnormally fast heart rhythms, such as atrial fibrillation and supraventricular tachycardia, which can often be treated naturally. Yet most people are only given a choice of either pharmaceuticals or ablation. Pharmaceuticals are usually ineffective, cause side effects, and may even increase the risk of death. Ablation involves the burning of heart tissue. Sounds barbaric, right? Yet this procedure is performed every day, all over the world.

For atrial fibrillation, ablation is 50% effective at best, and often requires a second procedure. Radiation exposure is immense as over one hour of fluoroscopy time is typically used. The doctor may burn a hole right through the heart, leading to a situation called cardiac tamponade. Now the patient has blood in the sac surrounding the heart, limiting blood flow. This blood needs to be drained ASAP, or the patient can die.

I am very successful at reducing atrial fibrillation and other heart rhythm problems in my patients. Chiropractic care, acupuncture, and yoga are all proven to help. Nutritional changes such as avoiding wheat, gluten, sugar, corn, dairy, and soy, and supplements like omega-3 fish oil, magnesium, vitamin C, E, and taurine all reduce atrial fibrillation. Getting more sleep and reducing stress levels reduces atrial fibrillation. Often, kicking the caffeine habit can cure the heart symptoms.

★**LIVE WELL**: Ablation poses risks that can lead to the patient's death, for only a small possible benefit.

DEFIBRILLATORS

A defibrillator, or "shock box," is an implanted metal device in the left, upper-chest region. A wire known as a lead is connected from the brains of the device (the generator) to the heart muscle. The device monitors the heart rhythm 24/7 and if it senses an unstable situation, can shock the heart back to normal and possibly save the person's life.

There are some conditions where implanting a defibrillator offers plenty of benefit. Of course there is risk, and risk has to be weighed against benefit. But most devices these days are placed in patients who never had a cardiac arrest or unstable heart rhythm. These are patients whose heart function is less than 35%. Among this population with below normal heart function, studies conclude defibrillators decrease the chance of dying by 7% over 5 years. In other words, 14 people get a device to save one life over five years; 13 people derive no benefit, yet get all the risk.[132] The problem is, we cannot identify the person whose life will be saved.

The risks of the procedure include death, respiratory failure, and cardiac tamponade. Infection is a possibility and the entire device may need to be removed along with a lengthy course of antibiotics. Removing the device can leave a hole in the heart. This is dangerous business. Patients often complain of discomfort at the insertion site for months, even years after the procedure. Seat belts and clothing can also be irritating. Lastly, unnecessary shocks can be an unpleasant surprise to the patient. Doctors rarely warn of this possibility, yet it is a frequent occurrence. My advice: Ask a lot of questions before a permanent device is installed into your body. The long-term effects of implanted foreign metals are still unknown.

★**LIVE WELL**: Common procedures like defibrillators are beneficial in some instances, but also carry considerable risk.

All this is tolerable if the device will save your life. But 1 out of 14 over five years? This is much better than statin data, or the supposed benefits from most drugs, but still it only represents a small chance of benefit. The question always remains: can natural therapies do better? Don't forget, the patients in these studies eat fast food and cupcakes, and drink soda pop. If we did a study where one group eats Paleo, takes proven supplements, exercises, reduces stress, and avoids chemicals, and the other group gets a defibrillator, who would live longer? This type of study will never be done. You be the judge.

★**LIVE WELL**: The Paleo Plan—ancestral nutrition, proven supplements, exercise, stress reduction, and avoidance of chemicals—is the solution.

ECG (EKG)

The electrocardiogram was invented over 100 years ago in Germany, hence the use of K instead of the C in English. (Just a little trivia.) This test is very inexpensive and does not put the patient at any risk. It is nice to check a baseline ECG to use for future comparison in case something happens and you wind up in the emergency room. I often advise people to carry a copy in their wallet. An ECG is also a quick screening test that can disclose certain conditions that could lead to bad outcomes.

CASE STUDY

Jeff was a 44-year-old male with hypertension and a family history of heart disease. He was a little overweight and had some shortness of breath with heavy exertion. A cardiologist had recommended a stress treadmill. During the stress test, he exercised for 14 minutes and stopped because he was getting "winded." The other parts of the test were normal, including his ECG tracing. But unfortunately, he was injected with the radioactive chemical technetium, an addition to the test that was totally unnecessary. Images obtained after exercise showed a mild defect at the tip of his heart. This was similar to the image before the exercise. Heart function was normal. Despite the blatantly low risk test, an angiogram was recommended.

Jeff came to see me to review his case, not wanting to undergo the same invasive test that led to his mother's stroke. It turned out Jeff had felt short of breath upon extreme exercise for quite some time. He did not complain of any chest pain. After reviewing his history and examining Jeff, I explained to him the angiogram was totally unnecessary. He did very well on his stress test and the abnormal scan (which was unnecessary, exposing him to dangerous radiation) was likely a false positive, meaning there was no actual blockage.

After a lengthy discussion with me, Jeff decided against the procedure. He listened to my advice and began following Paleo nutrition and did a chemical survey of his house. He pulled out the carpeting, changed to an eco-friendly laundry detergent, and stopped wearing cologne. Now, three years later, Jeff has never felt better; he lost 15 pounds, and recently did a rim-to-rim hike of the Grand Canyon.

ACTION PLAN

1. Avoid unnecessary testing.
2. Skip radiative tests whenever possible.
3. Seek another opinion.
4. If you are radiated, consume plenty of anti-oxidants before and after the procedure.
5. Ask the number needed to treat (NNT) for any drug or procedure. If the doc doesn't know, please ask them to find out for you.

Chapter 8

OUR TOXIC WORLD

"For the first time in the history of the world, every human is now subjected to contact with dangerous chemicals, from the moment of conception until death."
—Rachel Carson

This chapter is all about chemicals and what to do about them. In no way are the following pages meant to be all-inclusive of the poisonous environment in which we live. What I mean to highlight here are some of the major sources of toxins and some simple ways to get them out of our bodies and out of our lives. Keep your eyes open and question everything you put in or put on your body, store in your home, or share in your workspace and neighborhood. Run through your day from start to finish, and think about all of the toxins to which you are exposed. Get ready to protest the cell tower next to your home, or worse, next to your child's school (as happened to us just a few years ago, which is just one of the reasons we decided to homeschool).

In a study spearheaded by the Environmental Working Group (EWG.org), researchers found an average of 200 industrial chemicals and pollutants in the umbilical cord blood. Tests revealed a total of 287 different chemicals in the group. The umbilical cord blood of these 10 children, collected by the Red Cross after the cord was cut, harbored pesticides, consumer product ingredients, and wastes from burning coal, gasoline, and garbage. How sad to bring a baby into this toxic soup. Our two boys were born at home with a midwife. Heather painstakingly avoided chemicals and toxins during her pregnancies. Being born into a sea of pollution is not fair to our babies.

Early on my path to becoming a natural cardiologist I met with Doris Rapp MD. She is a research pioneer on how toxins destroy our health. Reading her books and watching her videos should be a requirement in all medical schools. It should be a requirement of every expecting parent, part of a curriculum called, "Do you know anything about how to be a good parent?" The Drs. Wolfson will create the educational program for our children, not the government, unless we want the sponsor to be Big Pharma, Big Tobacco, and Big Processed Food. Of course, *Silent Spring* by Rachel Carson is the original call to arms regarding chemicals and pesticides. Even before Carson was the earth-shattering book, *The Jungle*, by Upton Sinclair, which exposed the meat-packing industry in Chicago. Pesticides are a major health hazard as discussed in Chapters 3 and 4.

★LIVE WELL: Recommend a homebirth to family and friends. Greatest experience in the world for all parties involved.

POLLUTION

What we don't see can kill us. Actually, you can usually see pollution very clearly. On a sunny day, as you fly into a city or drive to a metropolitan area, you can see a brown cloud enveloping the sky. This toxic cloud is full of chemicals, destroying our health, and serving as a major cause in the increase of cancer, learning disorders, asthma, and many other diseases. How sad it is to live in a city such as Phoenix, LA, New York, or Chicago when the inhabitants are warned not to go outside because of air pollution. But the outdoors is not the only source of inhaled irritants; indoor air may be 10 times as bad, leaving our children in the most vulnerable position of all.

Air pollution is a major problem worldwide and is associated with an increased risk for cardiovascular disease. Air contains life-giving oxygen and nitrogen, but nowadays it also contains disturbingly toxic levels of carbon monoxide, ozone, sulfur dioxide, and thousands of types of particles, collectively known as particulate matter. We have known for years that air pollution causes lung disease, but its link to poor cardiovascular health is new on the radar screen. One again, the government is on the back of doctors preventing them from claiming a multivitamin is healthy, but sadly absent regarding our environment.

★**LIVE WELL**: Indoor air is more dangerous than outdoor air.

Where does this pollution come from? Well, look around. Check out the millions of automobiles and trucks on the road. Look at the cloud of dark fumes spit out of an exhaust pipe as a truck accelerates. Look at the factories and fuel plants that are polluting our world. Go outside and smell the toxic laundry products your neighbor is using, as the dryer exhaust is blown out of their house. Witness cigarette smoke releasing hundreds of chemicals into the air with each puff. FYI, the new E-cigs are probably not any better.

How about the new carpet, the new paint, the new cabinets, and the new car smell? Do you think these are natural fragrances? These are a tremendous source of cancer and heart disease. Candles, air fresheners, and cleaning agents are all chemicals that destroy our health. Do you get your car washed and the inside cleaned? Do you think the products used on the interior are natural? Think again (and bring your own next time). The pollutants are everywhere. Take note of every single thing in your house and its toxic potential. Before you buy anything, think about its possible health dangers. Get the toxins out of your home and your workspace.

The chemicals are breathed into our bodies through the lungs, absorbed through skin, and ingested from food and water. From these portals of entry, the toxins move into the blood stream and are recognized by the immune system as foreign invaders. This sets off the body's inflammatory response and ultimately leads to cardiovascular disease in forms such as atherosclerosis (blockages), hypertension, and heart rhythm problems.

★LIVE WELL: Change your life by changing your environment: get rid of the chemicals and pollutants in your home today.

Airborne particles are linked to heart attacks, stroke, atrial fibrillation, diabetes, and vascular diseases.[133] According to a report on the Global Burden of Disease, throughout the world particulate air pollution is estimated to cause 3.1 million deaths a year and 22% of disability adjusted life years (DALY) due to ischemic heart disease.[134] Recently, a study was published on air pollution in the *British Medical Journal*. The results were in line with previous reports demonstrating the more pollution in the air, the more cardiovascular events.[135] A recent Danish study came to a similar conclusion, with cardiovascular death rates the highest in those who experienced pollution and also consumed the least vegetables and fruit.[136] Could air pollution and chemicals lead to "idiopathic" cardiomyopathy, the supposedly unknown cause of a weakness in the heart muscle? It is only "unknown" to the doctors who do not know the right questions to ask, and who lack true medical education.

Ozone is a unique form of oxygen. This molecule is beneficial in the atmosphere as it protects us from excess solar radiation. The problem starts when ozone interacts with manmade pollutants. This combination is very dangerous, and according to the Environmental Protection Agency, is a cause of disease. Free radicals are formed, leading to inflammation and oxidative stress, with the end result being cardiovascular and lung diseases. Free radicals promote cancer and neurologic diseases such as dementia and Parkinson's. Studies exposing blood vessels to ozone found arterial damage and decreased ability of the artery to expand.[137] Ozone causes LDL particles to become oxidized (damaged), which you recall leads to their migration into arteries, ultimately causing coronary artery disease. As we destroy the environment, ground level ozone will increase as a health hazard.

★**LIVE WELL**: Exposure to ozone and other pollutants in the air weakens the heart's muscle tissue.

Studies confirm other air pollutants, such as nitrogen dioxide, carbon disulfide, and sulfur dioxide, are associated with an increased risk of heart attacks and sudden cardiac death. A 2014 study showed those people with the highest levels of POPS (persistent organic pollutants) had the worst blood tests.[138] Another 2014 study showed air pollution was a risk factor for heart attack and pulmonary embolism (blood clots in the lungs). Lead in polluted air is very toxic to the cardiovascular system, leading to hypertension, atherosclerosis, and heart enlargement. Carbon monoxide from cars and trucks, cigarette smoke, and the burning of fossil fuels competes with oxygen in our bodies to literally starve our cells.

A 2007 study, published in the prestigious *New England Journal of Medicine*, convinced 20 men with coronary artery disease to be exposed to diesel fumes. Compared to filtered air, diesel fumes led to evidence of myocardial ischemia (lack of oxygen to the heart) and caused a decrease in blood fibrinolytic enzymes, tiny "Pacmen" that dissolve blood clots. This is a unique study, which provided direct evidence of toxicity from air pollution.[139] Another study found diesel exhaust increases blood pressure.[140] Think about that the next time your car window is down while a dump truck or semi accelerates. Studies on the dangers of pollution appear very frequently these days. I think it is time to stop "studying" and start acting. Let's put the money and other resources toward stopping those who pollute our planet.

Do you ever wonder about the health of those who work curbside check-in at an airport? I think about these husbands, wives, mothers, and fathers sitting in carbon monoxide exhaust all day long. We have known for over 30 years that there is a risk to those who work at the Department of Motor Vehicles. Not only do they carry a higher cardiovascular risk, they are at an increased chance of developing cancer. In a sad example of irony, they are hired to prevent pollution from the very vehicles that are poisoning them to death.[141] Similarly, tunnel workers are at a much higher risk of cardiovascular disease while on the job.

Fortunately, the risk for these individuals starts to subside after a career change to a less toxic occupation.[142]

★**LIVE WELL**: Carbon monoxide and other pollutants compete with oxygen in the air. Remember this: No oxygen, no life.

Those who know The Drs. Wolfson recognize our number one passion and purpose is to protect children. The dangers of chemicals to children could fill an encyclopedia. A recent study discovered autism rates are doubled in children born in polluted areas. Those boys also had a 600% increase in genital malformations.[143] If we do not make the change for ourselves, we must for our children.

While writing this book, I saw a report from the World Health Organization (WHO) regarding air pollution. They estimate the annual death toll from pollution is over 7 million people per year worldwide. A large part of this stems from the fact so many people around the world use coal and fire for indoor heating and cooking. Yet millions of deaths can be attributed to outdoor pollution. Heart disease, stroke, lung disease, and lung cancer were deemed responsible for the vast majority of deaths according to the WHO report, but the real cause is the damage from poor nutrition and harmful chemicals.

★**LIVE WELL**: If only we could purchase bottled air as easily as we can clean water!

ACTION PLAN: START WITH WHAT YOU CAN CONTROL FIRST YOUR HOME

1. Get an air filtration system.[144] Do not allow anyone in your house who smells toxic. Do not permit anyone to smoke in your house. Make the addict go outside to smoke. All of these toxins stick to clothes, furniture, walls, etc. BY REPRIMANDING A TOXIC OFFENDER, YOU MAY SAVE THEIR LIFE.

2. Immediately get rid of all candles, air fresheners, and chemical sanitizers. Remove anything that produces an odor. All new patients in my office are reminded not to wear any scented skin or hair products.

3. Use natural laundry products and avoid the toxic laundry detergent, fabric softener, and dryer sheets. Check out brands like Seventh Generation and Dr. Bronner's Sal Suds. Use distilled white vinegar with your wash as a fabric softener, for preserving colors, and for static cling. If your old washer/dryer cannot be cleaned adequately with white vinegar, you may need to purchase a new set. Keep the washer door open between loads to prevent mold formation.

4. Get the carpet out and install wood floors without adhesives. Paint with zero VOC (volatile organic compounds) products. I painted my office with a milk-based paint. Smelled like a vanilla milkshake for a couple months.

5. Buy natural furniture without varnish or get used furniture that has already off-gassed. If something new smells, let it sit outside of your house until the smell is gone.

6. Open windows frequently because indoor air is usually worse than outdoor (unless your neighbor is mowing his lawn with a gas mower blowing fumes into your house).

7. Most products labeled as unscented still emit noxious chemicals. Example here is dryer sheets. Make sure you are buying natural items.

Try to make an impact at work. Show your boss this chapter and ask them to read it. I realize most people are not going to picket next to a coal plant or lay down in front of a diesel truck. Nonetheless, try to make an impact in the world and realize what is going on around us. If each person does his or her part, the world will become a better place.

★LIVE WELL: Take action at home and work to create a pollutant-free environment. Do it today.

SECOND HAND TOBACCO SMOKE

Unless you were living under a rock for 50 years, you know smoking causes heart and lung disease, cancer, and other harmful effects upon the human body. The Germans knew about the dangers of tobacco as early as the 1930s and banned smoking on buses and trains. Pregnant women were not allowed to smoke, and tobacco advertising was outlawed. Hitler (may he rot in hell) knew tobacco would hinder his plans for a perfect race. Contrast this to the U.S., which did not acknowledge tobacco dangers until the 1960's and made little effort to curtail its use until the 1980s. For years, a child could buy a pack of cigarettes in any vending machine. I know, because I was one of those kids.

Why doesn't our government ban smoking around children? Follow the money. The tax dollars from the tobacco industry can support a lot of pork-barrel spending. It is estimated that $25,000,000 per year is spent by tobacco lobbyists. (opensecrets.org).

According to the Center for Disease Control, secondhand smoke causes nearly 34,000 premature deaths from heart disease in the U.S. among nonsmokers. The risk of heart disease is increased by 25-30% for those exposed to second-hand smoke. The risk of stroke is also increased by 25-30%, leading to an additional 8,000 deaths per year. How many thousands more are incapacitated from cardiovascular disease due to secondhand smoke and don't die?[145] In 2013, data from a CT scan study found secondhand smoke doubles the risk of coronary calcification vs. non-exposed people.[146] Second-hand smoke is linked to hypertension, as noted by an increased risk of hypertension among flight attendants who breathed tobacco for hours at a time in a pressurized airborne tube.[147] Lung cancer and emphysema rates are much higher in people exposed to second-hand smoke. I said it before and I will say it again: if you smoke in front of a child, you are committing child abuse and should be punished to the full extent of the law.

★LIVE WELL: The health risks tobacco causes to non-smokers should make it illegal. Smoking around children should be illegal. Pregnant women should not be allowed to smoke.

What about third-hand smoke, defined as the chemical residue left on the clothing, furniture, and anything else where particles from cigarette smoke can adhere? Is there proof of cardiac effects? There is some animal data. Mice exposed to third-hand smoke showed alterations in multiple organs and carcinogens, similar to those found in children exposed to second-hand smoke. Lipid levels increased, as did the risk of fatty liver disease. Elevated markers of inflammation were also noted.[148] It turns out, dad smoking outside by himself is not so safe for the rest of the family because he brought the chemicals back in the house attached to his clothes. Patients point to a family history of illness, but it is all about them being exposed to the same toxins as their parents.

BISPHENOL A (BPA)

Do you drink out of plastic bottles? Do you ever wonder why the plastic bottle is labeled "do not refill?" You need to learn about the toxic effects of BPA. Bisphenol A (BPA) is a synthetic molecule used in the manufacture of plastics and in the epoxy resins lining food and beverage containers. It is one of the most produced chemicals in the world. BPA is classified as an endocrine disrupting chemical (EDC) because it interferes with hormones such as estrogen, testosterone, and others.

Most people harbor plastic in their body as evidenced from the detectable BPA metabolites in the urine of 80–90% of the population worldwide. Frighteningly, nine out of ten infants are born with detectable BPA in their body, according to the Environmental Working Group. The main source of exposure is through consumption of packaged food and beverages, with additional exposure from drinking water, shopping receipts, produce bags, personal care products, and inhalation of household dusts. In fact, a study published in *JAMA* in February 2014 showed BPA from paper receipts is easily absorbed through the skin.[149] Cashiers are at high risk for exposure. Aluminum cans contain a BPA lining. Disposable coffee cups are not made from paper alone, as common sense tells you they would leak if they were. The key to the integrity of the cup is often plastic. What do you think hot coffee does to plastic? Shampoos, laundry detergents, soaps, and even vitamin bottles typically contain BPA.

Even products labeled BPA-free are still made from synthetic compounds that get into our bodies. They may have worse possible effects than BPA. This is analogous to a vaccine manufacturer removing mercury from the shot, yet filling it with other chemicals. Pick your poison.

★**LIVE WELL:** Nearly nine out of ten people in the world carry traces of BPA in their blood and urine.

Multiple studies show an association between BPA in urine and cardiac disease. A recently published trial found the highest amount of BPA is associated with the most severe coronary artery disease.[150] BPA affects the heart by reducing nitric oxide (responsible for dilating vessels), altered vascular reactivity to endothelin-1 (vessel constrictor), oxidative stress (recruits damaged LDL to vessels), and inflammation. BPA also affects hormonal interaction with vascular smooth muscle and may interfere with cellular calcium channels. BPA has also been shown to induce diabetes in rabbits.

BPA falls into the category of Food Contact Materials, or FCM. Food comes in contact with packaging from the lid, the seal on the lid/container interface, and of course, the container itself. Do you think a milk carton is actually made of paper? What happens when water meets paper? The carton is a paper/plastic composite of unknown toxicity. Formaldehyde is often included in FCM. Among the over 4,000 known chemicals in product packing are tributyltin, triclosan, and phthalates. These are all linked to cancer, fertility issues, and neurologic disease. If you think some government agency is watching for your safety, think again.

Don't fret because you can reduce your exposure to plastic and other FCM easily and measurably. Here are a few proven suggestions:

- Never buy plastic water bottles and only drink out of glass.
- Rinse any food that came in contact with plastic (packaged meat etc.).
- Use cotton produce bags.
- Install under-sink water system with minimal plastic tubing or whole-house filtration.

- Avoid canned foods. If you do eat canned, make sure it is labeled BPA free
- Store food in glass containers.
- Make your nut (almond, coconut) milk fresh, not store-bought in BPA-lined cartons.
- Buy a quality air purifier.
- Open windows frequently.
- Use bar soap and minimize personal care products in plastic. Use organic soap.
- Buy natural children's toys and never let a child put plastic in their mouth, including most pacifiers.
- And of course, wash your hands before you eat.

ELECTROSMOG

In the course of human history, it is obvious we were never exposed to electricity. Our bodies are now crying out, "What is happening to me?," as they are constantly bathed in electrosmog. Electrosmog is the invisible pollution from electronic devices. Even when something is plugged in but not on, we are exposed.

The most common sources of electrosmog are:

- Mobile phones/cordless phones
- Cordless baby monitors (what does electrosmog do to a baby?)
- Mobile/cellular phone masts/towers/transmitters
- Wireless networks (turn it off at night)
- Microwave ovens
- Any electrical system with a power cord
- Smart meters- electric and water (Get them removed from your house.)

★LIVE WELL: Electrosmog, pollution from electronic devices, is a form of "invisible" pollution.

Cell phone towers are popping up like mushrooms in a garden. We pulled our son from a school where the flagpole was actually a cell tower in disguise—

on a preschool campus! Some disgusting people will do anything for money. Go to antennasearch.com to find the towers in your area.

What are the health effects to us and our children? Thousands of satellites in space send constant electromagnetic signals to earth. Don't ask me to show you evidence of danger: Prove to me it's safe. Smart meters are outside your house and allow the utility company to keep a close eye on your usage. This device shoots an electrical impulse into your house, right through concrete walls, and communicates with all your appliances. You wouldn't want to stand near a smart meter for too long. It's a catastrophe that the meter is usually outside of a bedroom, where the unassuming victim is sleeping.

Some of the electrosmog is absorbed into the body, causing an unknown amount of damage. The entire neurologic system relies on electricity to send signals from the brain all the way to the tip of the toes, and everything else in between. In fact, every cell in our body has a delicate balance of energy inside and outside of the cell. Can you imagine the subtle disruptions occurring trillions of times a second?

★**LIVE WELL**: Cell phone towers are becoming an "in your face" form of electrosmog.

If you had an ECG, you witnessed the electrical system of the heart in action. This simple test measures the electrical activity in the heart causing a heart contraction. There are plenty of studies[151] that demonstrate how electromagnetic fields EMF negatively affect the heart in ways such as:

1. Increased or decreased heart rate
2. Decreased heart rate variability
3. Increased arrhythmias
4. Increased heart cell free radicals
5. Decreased heart cell glutathione

Electrosmog may also cause:

- Headaches
- Disruptive sleep
- Chronic fatigue
- Depression
- Erratic blood pressure
- Skin complaints
- Unusual behavioral in children

Over the years I saw thousands of patients with abnormal heart rhythms ranging from skipped beats, to atrial fibrillation, to lethal heart rhythms such as ventricular tachycardia. Is it possible electrosmog is to blame? The heart is an electrical organ. It stands to reason that radiation from electric devices affects the electrical activity of our heart.

Recently, I was walking through Whole Foods and approached a woman who was carrying her cell phone in the left strap of her sports bra. The phone was literally sitting right on top of her heart. The conscientious physician I am, I approached the woman and advised her of the dangers and typical symptoms associated with EMF exposure. She was very grateful for my advice, told me she had experienced palpitations for years, and admitted doctors were not able to help with her symptoms. Some people are so sensitive they need to turn off the power to their bedroom, or even the entire house, to avoid symptoms of electrosmog; others must move to remote areas without cell phone towers or high-tension electrical wires.

★**LIVE WELL**: Your bedroom is a primary source of electrosmog in your home.

EVEN MORE CHEMICALS

Multiple studies confirm that chemicals wreak havoc on the cardiovascular system and the rest of the body. PFOA (perfluorooctanoic acid) is a synthetic chemical that makes water bead on a surface (doesn't allow water/liquids to penetrate clothing). It has been used in the manufacture of such prominent consumer goods as Teflon and Gore-Tex. Available since the 1940's, PFOA persists indefinitely in the environment and is carcinogenic in animals. It is detected in the blood of 98% of the US population, and at high levels in chemical plant employees and surrounding subpopulations. PFOA has been detected in industrial waste, stain-resistant carpets, carpet cleaning liquids, house dust, microwave popcorn bags, clothing, water, food, and cookware.

As recently reported in the *Annals of Internal Medicine*, researchers found people with high PFOA were more likely to suffer from hypertension and abnormal cholesterol. They also had the highest risk of coronary and peripheral artery disease.[152] PFOA has also been shown to increase the risk for diabetes[153] and lipid abnormalities in children.[154]

★LIVE WELL: Beware of the chemicals in such common household items such as carpets, carpet-cleaning liquids, microwave popcorn bags, clothing, water, food, and Teflon.

In 2012, a study was released that examined work-related exposure to chemicals and the incidence of cardiovascular disease. The exposed group consisted of 180 male workers chronically exposed to a mixture of organic solvents including styrene, toluene and xylene in plastic products and paint manufacturing factories; the control group comprised 135 male workers in machinery and metal product manufacturing factories who had not been exposed to those organic solvents or other hazardous chemicals. The purpose was to find similar people in the same industry who lived in the same area and led the same lifestyle. Not surprisingly, the exposed group had a much lower antioxidant capacity, setting up those workers for increased cardiovascular events.[155] Another study showed solvents increased blood pressure and were associated with fatty liver changes.[156] A case report from many years ago discussed a patient with an irregular heart rhythm related to the dry-cleaning agent PERC. His symptoms totally resolved when the exposure to PERC was removed.[157] Cancer and neurologic disease are also likely influenced by PERC. PERC is outlawed in new dry cleaning businesses, but the old-timers were grandfathered in. Lastly, "organic" dry-cleaners are a joke and are likely just as dangerous. The use of the word organic only applies to food.

If pesticides kill bugs and herbicides kill plants, those chemicals will kill us. Health issues related to these poisons have been known for years, and were the subject of Rachel Carson's shocker *Silent Spring*, published in 1962. Despite these alarms and calls to action, is anything changing? There is a huge body of evidence on the relation between exposure to pesticides and an elevated rate of cancer, diabetes, neurodegenerative disorders like Parkinson's, Alzheimer's, birth defects, and reproductive issues. There is also evidence pesticide exposure causes: respiratory problems, particularly asthma and chronic obstructive pulmonary disease (COPD), cardiovascular disease, chronic kidney disease, autoimmune diseases such as systemic lupus erythematous and rheumatoid arthritis, chronic fatigue syndrome, and aging. At the most basic level, pesticides, as well as other chemicals, affect the way cells function. They cause genetic damage, interfere with hormones, and damage the energy producing mitochondria.[158]

★**LIVE WELL**: If pesticides kill bugs and herbicides kill plants, those chemicals will kill you.

CASE STUDY

Angie W. came to see me as a young woman with migraine headaches and difficulty sleeping. After a thorough history, it became clear her problems began after moving into a recently remodeled house and sleeping on a new mattress. I explained to her that she was living in a toxic soup and something needed to change. I convinced her to get rid of the mattress loaded with chemicals such as flame-retardants and synthetic materials. After all, she was spending 10 hours a day on that mattress, mostly tossing and turning. She bought an organic mattress from Lifekind.com. I advised her to get an air purifier and leave her windows open during the day. Lastly, Angie removed all the electronic items from her bedroom except a lamp, which she unplugged before bed.

After two months Angie returned to my office as a new woman. She no longer suffered from migraines and was sleeping a solid eight hours without interruption. Her energy was back, and her allergies were gone. As an added bonus, Angie glowed from delight about the "bun in the oven." This is what the profession of doctor and healer is all about.

ACTION PLAN

1. Avoid outdoor pollution when possible.
2. Do not consume food or beverages from plastic or cans.
3. Don't smoke or be around those who do.
4. Say no to chemicals found in personal-care products.
5. Minimize electronic devices, especially in the bedroom and on your body (buyer beware about devices/gadgets that claim to minimize EMF exposure).
6. Unplug your microwave. Never use Teflon-coated or aluminum pots and pans.
7. Get the smart meter removed from your house.
8. Don't dry clean your clothes.
9. Wear cotton clothing that can be washed and ironed.
10. Stop spraying pesticides and herbicides. You are destroying our planet!

Chapter 9

HEAVY METAL MADNESS

"Look deep into nature, then you will understand everything better."
—Albert Einstein

I f I mention heavy metals, those words likely conjure up big hair bands like Bon Jovi and Aerosmith. In this case, I am referring to a loosely defined group of metallic elements such as lead, aluminum, mercury, cadmium, and arsenic. The path to good health is unfortunately littered with these toxins and medical doctors are absolutely clueless regarding their dangers. Your standard medical doctors do not know what to do with elevated body metals. Read on and you will learn how we are exposed, what the typical symptoms are, and what to do about it.

Remember back in high school when you stared with a blank face at the periodic table? That chart represents the basic elements or atoms, which encompass so much of what we discuss in medicine—sodium, potassium, zinc, etc. In fact, there are over 100 different elements. Heavy metals are elements naturally occurring in the earth's crust, but because of manmade pollution they invaded our ecosystem. The sources of human exposure to heavy metals creates a long list: coal and other fossil fuels, dental fillings, vaccinations, fertilizers, food processing, contaminated water, tobacco, body care products, canned goods, etc. In fact, rice and chicken are a significant source of arsenic, even if they are organic.

Mercury, aluminum, and lead do not play a role in the health or function of the human body. They are not part of any natural process in any organ or structure. The toxicity of heavy metals in the body can lead to blockage of enzymes, impairing antioxidants, and increasing oxidative stress.[159] All of this culminates in the symptoms we call disease. Once again, find the CAUSE to get the CURE.

Basically, the presence of metals is like putting a crowbar into the spokes of a wheel. In this case, wheels are enzyme pathways in the body where protein A is converted to protein B. Lead, for example, blocks the ability of magnesium to do its job. Heavy metals also lead to the formation of free radicals, which can damage DNA and lipids such as LDL, and ultimately destroy glutathione, the main antioxidant of the body. If you are not making glutathione, you can say hello to disease. Glutathione is easily tested from Spectracell and other companies commonly used in my practice.

Every person has a different level of tolerance to all toxins, including heavy metals, based on genetics, nutritional status, and the total body burden of other chemicals. Testing of heavy metals in the body can be done in many different ways, including serum, hair, urine, and even through cells. Each method has its pro's and con's. Let's take a deeper look at the most common metals, remembering that over a dozen can be tested, and are likely to interfere with optimal health and lead to high blood pressure, strokes, heart attacks, cancer, and other health complications.[160]

★**LIVE WELL**: Heavy metals occur naturally in the earth's crust, but because of pollution and man-made products they invaded our ecosystem and our bodies.

LEAD

Whether you lived in Ancient Rome, or in today's society, lead was and still is a source of disease. The Roman water system used lead pipes and its toxicity was soon realized. Today lead is found all over the environment. Lead paint and leaded gasoline were major sources of contamination now outlawed in the U.S., but the effects are still present today. The combustion of leaded gas rained down on the earth to cause soil pollution from which there is no recovery. The lead will never go away. Lead is still found in many toys, burning fossil fuels, ammunition, and batteries. I test for lead in many patients and EVERYONE has detectable levels. This is why I feel everyone should take an oral chelator daily (more on this in a few pages).

If your blood pressure is high, it may be a lead issue. Studies correlate serum lead with an increased risk for hypertension. Lead may cause hypertension by interfering with nitric oxide availability and increasing renin and angiotensin production. Lead also interferes with the action of calcium, a nutrient highly involved with blood pressure regulation (and hundreds of other bodily functions). To the cells and molecules of the body, lead actually looks very similar to magnesium and potassium, thus interfering with both of these life-giving elements. If magnesium and potassium can't get to where they work, health problems will develop. A key will not fit in a lock if there is gum in it. Your body does not have a pharmaceutical deficiency causing high blood pressure, but instead may suffer complications due to lead.

★LIVE WELL: Lead is in everyone's body and can contribute to high blood pressure.

Chronic lead exposure may affect lipid metabolism and oxidative stress, and has been linked to atherosclerosis and increased cardiovascular mortality in humans. We know from animal studies, lead exposure promotes atherosclerosis. Elevated inflammatory markers such as hs-CRP are associated with elevated lead. The higher the CRP (C-reactive protein), the higher a person's risk of heart disease. Elevated lead is associated with a higher amount of homocysteine, the amino acid found in those with heart disease, blood clots, cancer, and dementia. Are you getting the picture? When it comes to heart health, lead is a nasty player.[161]

An interesting fact is blood pressure in women tends to increase after menopause. Could one factor leading to hypertension in these women be elevated lead floating around the body? You see, lead is stored in bone. As the osteoporotic bones weaken in menopausal women, lead is released and interferes with bodily function. These same women have an increased heart attack risk, possibly from the lead exposure. Osteoporosis is prevented by Paleo nutrition, staying physically active, and taking quality supplements.

★LIVE WELL: Lead is a likely contributor to the increase of hypertension among women during menopause.

Near and dear to me is the fact lead causes neurologic disease. Since my father died from the brain disorder Progressive Supranuclear Palsy, lead is something I do not want in my body, so I do my best to keep it out. This metal is a well-known cause of dementia such as Alzheimer's disease. Lead also damages the brain of developing infants and is a well-known cause of learning disabilities. The higher the lead in the brain, the lower the IQ. Lead is a causative factor for ALS (Amyotrophic Lateral Sclerosis, better known as Lou Gehrig's disease) and Parkinson's disease. Regrettably, it did not occur to me or other doctors to test my dad for heavy metals. In the days of his sickness, I was a typical medical doctor looking for the magic pill to fix him.

ALUMINUM

Aluminum is a relatively soft, durable, lightweight metal. Hundreds of uses are found in modern society. The number one exposure is likely aluminum in cookware. Your pots and pans may say stainless steel or copper, but they are loaded with aluminum. "Tin foil" is aluminum and can contaminate your food. Don't use it. Baking powder and food coloring contain aluminum, two ingredients found in most packaged goods. Aluminum is the key element in antiperspirants, and is tragically added to most vaccines that are injected into newborn babies. Just the exposure from soda cans alone is enough to spark a worldwide pandemic of disease. But did you realize this metal causes heart disease?[162]

A few years ago, coronary artery disease risk was studied in an aluminum smelting company employing over 6,000 men. Results from this study showed white-collar workers had HALF the risk of heart disease compared to blue-collar workers, the group actually exposed to the aluminum. The white-collar guys sit in meetings or behind a desk all day and are therefore less exposed to the aluminum in the plant. We can surmise that both groups would be at higher risk than the general population.[163] Smelting is a process that separates metal from the rock in which it was found. This way the metal can be purified and used for more buildings, more cars, and more vaccines. A 2014 study showed a 50% increase in the risk of cardiac events (heart attack, stroke, heart failure) amongst aluminum workers compared to the general population.[164] Aluminum has been implicated as a cause for Alzheimer's dementia and osteoporosis.[165] Is it possible aluminum-based antiperspirants applied to the armpits of most people cause breast cancer? Instances of men with breast cancer are exploding.

★**LIVE WELL**: Aluminum is a metal you should avoid, even under your arms, despite what the person next to you may think.

MERCURY

Mercury is a metal element that is liquid at room temperature. Ask most seniors about mercury and they will tell you stories about how they played with this metal as children (known then as quicksilver) during science class. That was a big mistake. I distinctly remember my high school chemistry teacher with a horrible tremor. Was it possible this came from frequent exposure to mercury? The "Mad Hatters" of England became famous as brain damaged individuals because of their exposure to mercury in the hat-making industry.

The main source of mercury pollution is from coal burning. Gold production accounts for 11% of emissions, so think about that the next time you want a piece of jewelry. Mercury contaminates our soil and water, and even many household items. Sadly, the oceans are loaded with pollutants, which concentrate in the larger fish of the food chain. Hence, never eat swordfish, tuna, shark, or other large fish. Mercury was used in glass thermometers and sphygmomanometers (blood pressure cuffs) as elemental mercury, and is still used in dental amalgam fillings. Organic mercury is found mainly in fish as methylmercury and in some vaccines as ethylmercury (thimerosal). In fact, many flu shot formulations contains billions of mercury atoms. Can you imagine the damage those billions of mercury atoms can do? Unfortunately, mercury is present in most light bulbs. At best, the public water system removes only 90% of mercury from waste water. The rest finds its way back into tap water and rivers, lakes, and streams.

★**LIVE WELL**: Mercury contaminates fish, water, soil, and even our light bulbs.

Years ago, thermometer and blood pressure cuff makers abandoned the use of this toxic element for safety reasons, but most of the dental industry and vaccine makers still feel it is safe to put in your body. If a fluorescent light bulb breaks, according to the Environmental Protection Agency, you must follow many steps for proper disposal. In fact, the EPA has a 76-page document intended for dentists as a guideline to develop an environmentally friendly practice on the disposal of mercury waste. The disposal of metal amalgams is serious business. Yet doctors apparently feel it is okay to put this very same mercury into your mouth or inject it into your blood stream. It appears the only safe place for mercury is in the human body. Do you see the lunacy in all this?

★**LIVE WELL**: Despite what your doctor may say, mercury does not belong in your body.

Mercury exposure has been shown to promote atherosclerosis. A great example of this is the fact dentists are at a higher heart attack risk than other populations. They breathe in mercury vapor all day implanting and replacing metal amalgams. The high mercury content of fish may diminish some of the beneficial effects of seafood on cardiovascular health. Some studies found a higher incidence of hypertension and diabetes in those people with elevated mercury. There is good reason pregnant women are advised against eating tuna.

We only recommend eating wild salmon, anchovies, and sardines. As discussed in Chapter 3, take chlorella after eating any seafood. Heather and I formulated a product named Cardio Superfood that contains chlorella and spirulina. More on these foods in Chapter 16.

Mercury can bind to glutathione, the antioxidant that plays a critical role in regenerating vitamins C and E. This leads to damage of molecules including lipids, which are then more likely to cause vessel plaque and blockages. Mercury damages the mitochondria, the tiny furnaces in every cell that are critical for energy production and suppresses nitric oxide production, the main dilator of arteries. Lastly, mercury disrupts blood clotting by interfering with platelets. This is a nasty particle and you should think twice about implanting it into your own, or your children's, bodies.

★**LIVE WELL**: Mercury levels in fish can make you rethink its role in your diet.

ARSENIC

Arsenic is the poison you hear about on the news when one person in a relationship wants to get rid of the other . . . permanently. High doses can kill people very quickly. But for the purpose of this book, we are talking about a chronic, low-level intake. Contaminated drinking water is the number one source of arsenic exposure worldwide. Chickens and pigs are high in this metal, as their feed often contains added arsenic to induce weight gain, improve color, and kill parasites. Our friends at Big Pharma are often involved in feed production. Although organic chicken contains some arsenic, the levels are much lower than conventional tortured fowl. Rice is another significant food source of exposure to arsenic, given the fact ground-water is loaded with arsenic and the rice avidly soaks it all up. Incidentally, cooking does not diminish the levels of any heavy metal, but rinsing the rice before cooking may help. Anyway, rice is not Paleo.

Coronary artery disease is more common in subjects with arsenic exposure from drinking water as compared to control subjects.[166] Similarly, hypertension is more common among residents in areas with high arsenic levels compared to those who experience low exposure. Arsenic from drinking water is also associated with an increased risk of developing type-2 diabetes mellitus, carotid artery disease, and stroke.[167] In Chile, deaths from heart attacks increased following a period of arsenic exposure in drinking water. Heart attack rates decreased after the source of the arsenic was removed. Likewise in southwestern Taiwan, mortality rates from heart disease declined after stopping the use of high arsenic well water. [168]

★LIVE WELL: Cooking does not eliminate metals like arsenic in food products.

How does arsenic inflict such damage on the cardiovascular system? It appears this toxic metal can interfere with the ability of a blood vessel to expand (dilate) or contract (constrict). Arsenic likely damages an enzyme called endothelial nitric oxide synthase (eNOS). This enzyme produces nitric oxide, which is the main dilator of blood vessels. If you have ever seen someone put a nitroglycerin tablet under their tongue, it is for the purpose of treating chest pain by increasing heart artery flow.

Similar to lead, high arsenic levels are associated with elevated homocysteine, the molecule seen in patients with hypertension, coronary artery disease (CAD), blood clots, and dementia. The detoxification of arsenic by the liver depletes B vitamins, so they are unavailable to process homocysteine, thus leading to its elevation. One solution is to make sure you take plenty of methylated B vitamins. Lastly, arsenic is a known carcinogen, meaning it causes cancers of the skin, liver, lung, bladder, etc.

How often do cardiologists check arsenic levels in patients with chest pain, hypertension, or heart disease? Just about never. Cardiologists could care less about metals and other toxins. There are no drugs to treat metals and no tests to order that can make money for the doctor. What if we avoided arsenic, other metals, and other toxins? What if we all ate Paleo? It is possible we would no longer need cardiologists.

★LIVE WELL: Arsenic consumes large amounts of vitamin B from the body, and can lead to cancer and heart disease, yet its presence in the body is rarely checked by cardiologists.

CADMIUM

Cadmium is a metal similar to zinc, but whereas the latter is healthy, the former is not and has no biological function. Smokers contain approximately twice the cadmium in their bodies as nonsmokers because tobacco soaks up this metal from the soil and fertilizers. Those exposed to second-hand smoke also suffer from cadmium toxicity. Over the years, cadmium has been used in batteries and metal products. The air and soil of the earth where our children play are contaminated from mining and pollution. Our food and water supply contain cadmium due to its use in fertilizers, herbicides, and pesticides.

Chronic cadmium exposure is associated with hypertension and diabetes.[169] It appears to promote atherosclerosis, and was independently associated with myocardial infarction and increased thickening of the blood vessel wall as estimated by intima-media thickness ratio.[170] This metal may wreak havoc by interfering with cellular calcium channels, leading to heart and blood vessel problems. Cadmium is a direct vasoconstrictor and inhibits vasodilator substances such as nitric oxide. Cadmium depletes the body of the antioxidant glutathione. Supplements to boost glutathione are frequently recommended in my practice. Unfortunately, it is hard to get this cadmium out of the body, even with chelation. Chlorella, fresh garlic, and garlic supplements are your best ways to rid your body of cadmium (more on chlorella and garlic in Chapter 16).

★**LIVE WELL**: Chlorella and garlic are heart healthy.

OTHER METALS

The above heavy metals are not the only ones to worry about. Tin, tungsten, thallium, thorium, antimony, barium, and gadolinium are just a few of the elements on the periodic table found in the blood where they do not belong. Barium is detected very often in blood and urine testing for heavy metals. How does barium get in your body? In the air we breathe. Have you ever had an MRI? The gadolinium is likely still floating around your body. Look at the fumes coming from a diesel truck, a local factory, or pictures from the Beijing Olympics. This exhaust is loaded with metals with no known function in human physiology. Research is limited, but the adverse effects on health are virtually limitless.

★**LIVE WELL**: The health consequences of heavy metals are limitless.

How do I know if I am high in metals?

There are many different ways to identify metals in the body. First off, you can do a blood test, but unfortunately this only reflects recent exposure. Go out for sushi one night and your mercury level will be high. I prefer the blood test that looks at intracellular metals in a red cell. This tells us what is in the bone marrow, the place where red cells are born. If levels are high in the bones, they are high in other organs, including the heart, blood vessels, and brain.

For years, doctors checked hair samples for metals, but what if the problem is simply your body doesn't excrete metals well? Mercury may not show up in your hair, but it could still be in your brain. Clearly, if your hair samples are high, you are toxic. This highlights an important fact: if any method of testing comes back elevated, you are definitely harboring toxic metals. On the other hand, just because a test is negative does not mean you are safe.

The diagnostic test of choice for body metal burden by most holistic doctors is urinalysis. Typically, a 24-hour urine is performed to assess metal levels, followed by a provocative agent or chelator. A chelator helps to remove heavy metals from the body. This agent can be DMSA, EDTA, or DMPS, short abbreviations for long chemical names. Once this is given, urine is collected for another 6-24 hours. The doctor then compares the pre- to post-metal levels to determine your body "burden." If you release a significant amount of metals after a chelator, you would do well to continue with chelation, especially if you suffer symptoms of metal toxicity.

★**LIVE WELL**: Chelate for symptoms that may be related to metal overload. Arterial blockage could be one of those indications.

WHAT TO DO ABOUT METALS

If you are diagnosed with high metal levels, the first thing you need to do is reduce exposure. You need to learn about each metal and find out where and when you were exposed. Look back to your childhood, your work history, places where you lived, etc. Think about your current exposure in your house and in your workplace. You, the patient, must be your own advocate to find the source. No one cares as much as you do. This includes paints, cookware, makeup, and laundry products. Your healthcare provider should be able to assist you on this quest.

Once the house is done, clean up your work place. There is not much you can do if you work as a miner or in a metal foundry, but the rest of us must strive to make an impact. When I toiled away in the hospital, I tried to get the custodial department to use non-toxic cleaning products. Vote with your wallet. Do not support corporations that manufacture or use poisonous materials.

If your mouth contains metal amalgams, a qualified holistic dentist must remove them. Do not ask your average mouth jockey for their opinion. In sheer denial, those docs refuse to believe they are poisoning their patients. There are excellent YouTube videos on the do's and don'ts of amalgam extraction. Next, avoid vaccinations that are loaded with metals. Swallowing metals in food or water gives your body a chance to not absorb the toxins. Injecting metals and other chemicals directly into your body defeats all natural defenses.

The best way to get toxins out of our bodies is through regular bowel movements and a high urine volume. Ideally, we should move our bowels like a dog does, 2-3x per day. Lots of fiber and fluids should ensure we achieve this goal. Drink quality, clean water at an amount equal to half your body weight in ounces. For example, a 150-pound person should drink at least 75 ounces daily. That is roughly 2½ quarts.

Another amazing way to get metals out of our bodies is through sweat. Whether through exercise or in a sauna, sweat is proven to contain metals. As this book was going to print, a study came out in JAMA: Internal Medicine that found a 63% lower chance of cardiac death in males who used a sauna daily! My wife's grandfather is 95 years old. His diet was always poor and he was exposed to just about every chemical possible, much of it during his military service. My wife believes he is alive because of years of playing tennis in the hot Florida sun working up a shirt-soaking sweat. Hot yoga is a great detox, and you will sweat buckets. But please check the work out environment to make sure toxins are not flowing back in. I performed hot yoga at a studio using toxic laundry detergents, and with wood floors that off-gassed glue at high temperatures. It defeated the whole purpose of the sweat.

> ★**LIVE WELL**: Get the metals and other toxins out of your body through regular bowel movements, plenty of urine, and lots of sweat.

CHELATORS

The word chelate comes from the Greek word for "claw." A chelator is any type of molecule that can claw onto or bind a metallic element, allowing it to be excreted by the body. The Food and Drug Administration recognizes certain chelating agents in the case of acute poisoning or an iron and copper overload. After all, chelators were developed during World War I to combat chemical warfare.

My first choice to bind metals and reduce body burden is the amazing food, chlorella. In addition to the plethora of health benefits belonging to this blue-green algae, such as phytonutrients and protein, chlorella has the ability to bind metals and increase their excretion. Animal studies confirm chlorella can bind to mercury and cadmium and get them out of the body.[171]

> ★**LIVE WELL**: Chelators like chlorella attach to metal and assist the body in excreting this toxic substance.

Another chelating option is zeolite, a volcanic ash that may help with metal burden. It has been used for decades to remove metals from wastewater. Zeolite has a high affinity for positively charged ions, such as mercury, lead, arsenic, and cadmium. Be careful though, zeolite can bind beneficial ions such as calcium, potassium, zinc, and magnesium. Ideally, zeolite should be used under medical supervision.

In the news recently are chelators such as EDTA and DMSA. These products were under a lot of scrutiny since the late 1980s after several patients died from their use. These isolated cases should not invalidate chelation; however, these incidents caused medical societies to develop protocols for appropriate use of chelators. Many doctors continue to use intravenous (IV) chelation for conditions ranging from cardiovascular disease to children with autism. Safety does not appear to be a concern when IV chelation is performed by experienced physicians.

Some doctors, myself included, are proponents of oral chelation using EDTA and DMSA. The premise is that everyone is toxic and exposed on a daily basis; therefore, we should chelate every day. These agents appear to be safe and are proven effective in eliminating metals. In fact, hundreds of studies back up the practice of oral chelation.

The groundbreaking TACT trial made headlines in 2013. This study looked at over 1700 patients with a history of a heart attack. Patients were divided into two groups: those who received EDTA IV chelation and those given an IV placebo. The results demonstrated an 18% reduction in cardiovascular events, including mortality, heart attack, stroke, and revascularization. The largest benefit was noted in people with a history of an anterior (front) infarction of their heart.[172]

Don't run out to your cardiologist for this type of treatment just yet. The trial was met with skepticism and debate. Medical doctors are very stubborn and refuse to give up on their antiquated Band-Aid treatments for heart disease, like statins and stents. We can only hope more data comes to light showing the benefit of getting the metal out of our bodies. In the meantime, check with your natural doctor about chelation.

★LIVE WELL: Oral chelation every day may be the best approach to getting the metal out of our bodies.

VACCINE DANGERS

The U.S. vaccine schedule calls for 69 vaccines by the time the child is 18 years of age. The long-term effects of the massive vaccination campaign are unknown, and there are few studies documenting vaccine safety. Big Pharma is frantically trying to create more vaccines for every ailment. Imagine the financial windfall for Big Pharma as medical societies recommend dozens of vaccines to children and adults. We are talking about billions of dollars here. All to combat diseases like the chicken pox (benign childhood disease). Humans evolved over millions of years without chemical injections. Do doctors think they can improve on Mother Nature?

Flu shots are recommended yearly, yet rarely work because viruses mutate. Vaccine manufacturers use last year's viruses, which miss the target. I think getting the flu is actually okay and may be beneficial. Sure, you lay in bed for a couple days feeling lousy, but it makes for a great cleanse/detox. You sweat and don't eat much, giving your gastrointestinal tract a rest. Don't let the scare tactics run your life. I worked in the hospital for 18 years. Death was rare from the flu, and was always in a person who had a long history of illness. Remember the Swine Flu, Bird Flu, and SARS? Those viruses were supposed to kill millions of people, yet suddenly disappeared. In 2014, it was all about Ebola. The US government is investing billions combating this bug. Yet, it has been around since the 1970's and people rarely die from it, IN Africa. That area has poor sanitation, poor food quality, and dirty water along with antiquated medical care. In developed nations, people will not be dropping like flies from Ebola. Don't get caught up in the hype, eat healthy and avoid chemicals to avoid disease. Be under the care of a natural doctor to get the best vitamins and intravenous therapy to boost your immune system.

In Chapter 10, "The Body Fights Back," I discuss the link between immune stimulation and cardiovascular disease. This is exactly what vaccines are designed to do, ramp up immune cells. Once again, there is no telling what this will do in the long run. We know of plenty side effects like fever, kidney failure, nervous system failure, and Stevens-Johnson Syndrome (a situation where third-degree burns form all over the body). Google images of Stevens-Johnson and you will be mortified.

★**LIVE WELL**: Receiving 70 vaccines by age 18 may not be the best thing for our hearts.

Check out the "other" ingredients in vaccines such as aluminum, mercury, formaldehyde, polyethylene glycol, and monosodium glutamate (MSG). The vaccines are grown on a medium such as human embryo cells, aborted fetal tissue, and animal proteins. I doubt these were healthy animals, and aborted fetal tissue does not sound like something I want injected into my body (or my child's). Yet this is what is happening to children 69 times by age 18. Do not believe for one second any researcher knows this is safe. Chemicals are never safe. Lastly, Hepatitis B is a virus contracted through intravenous drug use or sleeping with prostitutes. As my wife points out, the fact the Hep B vaccine is given to newborn babies should cause us to question the entire vaccine industry.

Paleo Nutrition and chemical avoidance are the way to health, not pharmaceuticals and vaccines. It is okay to catch a cold or the flu once in a while; that is the purpose of our immune system. These infections make our immune system stronger and ready for the next battle.

★**LIVE WELL**: Paleo nutrition and chemical avoidance is the best medicine.

CASE STUDY

Margaret was a 61-year old female who came to see me because her blood markers of inflammation were elevated. She also admitted to poor memory and "brain fog." Her primary care doctor wanted to prescribe a statin for an elevated hs-CRP. I explained to Maggy something was causing the inflammation and we needed to find out the CAUSE. I performed two tests on her, a food sensitivity panel and an intracellular heavy metal test. It turned out she was highly sensitive to dairy and soy. She was also very high in mercury and aluminum. Next we discussed her exposure to these metals and determined sushi (mercury), soda pop (aluminum cans), and cookware were the likely culprits.

Maggy gave up all dairy and soy products. She stopped eating sushi and drinking soda. At my recommendation, she purchased stainless steel cookware from SaladMaster. Because aluminum is found in many vaccines, I advised her against any further shots. I recommended she consume plenty of chelators like chlorella, garlic, and zeolite. She moved her bowels daily and drank plenty of clean water. Three months later, we repeated her blood inflammation test and were elated it was in the normal range. One year later, an assessment of metals revealed her levels of mercury and aluminum were much lower. Her daughter felt her memory was back to normal and the brain fog was gone.

ACTION PLAN

1. Avoid sources of heavy metals, especially cookware.
2. Get tested by a natural doctor skilled in the detection of metals.
3. Make sure you are flushing out your system by urinating, moving your bowels, and sweating.
4. Take chlorella every day, and certainly after a seafood meal.
5. Check out Zeolite.
6. Get your amalgams removed by a holistic dentist.
7. Consider oral or intravenous chelation.

Chapter 10

THE BODY FIGHTS BACK

"I arise in the morning torn between a desire to improve the world and a desire to enjoy the world. This makes it hard to plan the day."
—E. B. White

Doctors are great at creating a label for a constellation of symptoms and calling it a disease. For example, Parkinson's disease is abnormal walking, with diminished facial movement, rigidity of muscles, and tremors. Lupus is a set of over ten signs and symptoms to meet criteria for this diagnosis. Congestive heart failure is shortness of breath and swelling of the legs. Over the years, doctors identified groups of complaints and signs of illness, arrogantly tagging their last name to them. However, names do not tell us the cause, they only provide a label. Poor nutrition and chemicals are the CAUSE. Sickness is from too much of a bad thing or not enough of a good thing—excess or deficiency.

In between the cause and the label are inflammation, oxidative stress, and immune overstimulation. This concept comes from Mark Houston M.D., in his book, *What Your Doctor May Not Tell You About Heart Disease.* Dr. Houston teaches that the body only has these three finite responses to an infinite number of insults. Grasping this idea will improve your understanding of why nutrition and supplements work and why toxins are harmful. This chapter can get pretty technical so hang in there.

> ★LIVE WELL: Sickness is caused by too much of a bad thing,
> or not enough of a good thing.

The body is constantly working to maintain proper organ and cellular function. It does this by producing good molecules to counteract the bad ones, which cause cellular damage in the mitochondria, the energy factory found in nearly all of our cells. Lousy food, chemicals, metals, poor mental health, and physical inactivity lead to the production of potentially harmful players known as free radicals. Left unchecked, the free radicals will lead to decreased cellular function and eventual death. Solution: give your body the fuel it needs to defeat the bad guys.

INFLAMMATION

Do you suffer from chronic pain? That is a symptom of inflammation at work. Inflammation comes from the Latin root, inflamma, which means to ignite. Inflammation in your body is equivalent to your body being on fire. It is found in heart disease, cancer, diabetes, or Alzheimer's. You can tell if you are on fire from the most common complaint of all: PAIN. Pain is the number one reason a person goes to the doctor. The vast majority of adults suffer from pain somewhere in their body, and the vast majority of adults have evidence of cardiovascular disease. The more pain, the higher the risk of cardiovascular disease. 99.9% percent of doctors would never equate a sore back to heart attacks risk. When I see a patient in my office for consultation, I ask them to rate their overall pain from 1-10, with 10 being the worst. This includes chest pain, back pain, headaches, muscle discomfort, abdominal pain, and everything else that can ache. Invariably, the score is at least a 5 and often a 9 or 10. When I hear of pain in any area of the body, I think heart risk.

★**LIVE WELL**: Inflammation, body pain, and heart disease go hand in hand.

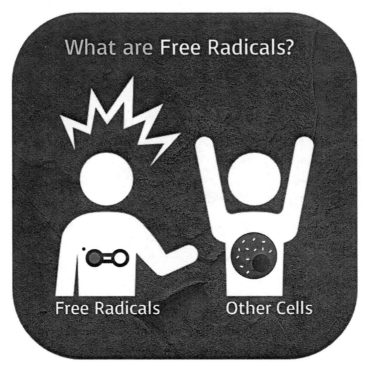

Free radicals are like robbers which are deficient in energy. They attack and snatch energy from other cells to satisfy themselves.

Chronic pain always goes hand in hand with inflammation. Inflammation can be a good thing. It helps to fight off infections by destroying bacteria and attracting cells to repair injured areas. This natural response is critical in the healing process of damaged tissue, whether from a paper cut or a broken leg. But these examples represent the short-term healing response, which is beneficial, as opposed to the chronic or long-term inflammation, which is very dangerous, stoking symptoms of disease. The worst situation may be when inflammation does not cause pain. We may not seek out a physician or get the appropriate diagnostic tests if we are not symptomatic. Elevated inflammation markers on a blood test should be taken very seriously.

SOUND THE ALARMS

Cytokines are tiny messengers produced from areas of inflammation by immune cells. These cells, such as macrophages, monocytes, and lymphocytes, release cytokines to signal other immune cells and molecules to come to the area in need. It's like a bugle call to rally the troops. These messengers, with names like interleukin (IL), tumor necrosis factor (TNF), and interferon, are easily tested by most commercial laboratories. The higher their levels, the more inflammation present, and the more cardiovascular risk. Is your doctor testing you for these dangerous messengers?

How Blockages Form

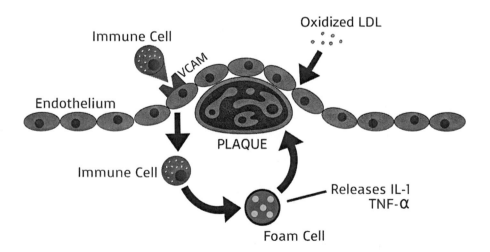

HOW CORONARY ARTERY BLOCKAGES FORM

Endothelial cells line blood vessels and are the barrier between the blood stream and the blood vessel. A healthy endothelium keeps unwanted items out, produces vasodilating molecules, which keep the vessels open, and allows the outer portion of the vessel to function normally. If we eat bad food or are exposed to chemicals, the endothelium becomes "leaky." This will allow unwanted molecules to traverse from the blood into the artery wall. This is how people get coronary artery disease. This is not actually a disease, but rather a response to damage done from toxins. Once again, a disease is just a label distracting us from the real cause. LDL particles, usually of the smaller, damaging variety, cross what should be a very selective endothelial barrier. A vicious cycle develops when immune cells respond to the damage and release cytokine messengers, which in turn recruit more immune cells. The culmination of this event is either a healed blockage (a stable plaque) or an unhealed blockage (unstable plaque). Stable can cause symptoms such as chest discomfort with exertion or shortness of breath; unstable can break loose, leading to a heart attack and possibly death.

> ★**LIVE WELL**: The natural response of the body is always to heal.

Read this slowly because it is somewhat technical: There is a protein called VCAM, which stands for vascular cell adhesion molecule. VCAM is like a little catcher's mitt on the surface of a blood vessel cell (see drawing above). These mitts catch immune cells like monocytes and lymphocytes, pulling them into the damaged area. The genes that make the VCAM proteins are activated by the messengers TNF-alpha and IL-1, both produced from existing immune cells. This is all part of the way the body heals the damaged blood vessel, leading to a blockage, which is really just a scar. Most labs will test for both TNF-alpha and IL-1. Cool stuff, huh?

> ★**LIVE WELL**: A blocked artery is similar to a scar on the skin. The scar didn't damage the area, it is a response to damage. Don't damage yourself.

Two tests historically used to determine levels of inflammation are the ESR and CRP. The human body does not make mistakes and CRP is made for a reason. Any time there is tissue damage, CRP is released from the liver and travels to the injured area to assist in cleanup and repair. A better test, known as hs-CRP, is highly correlated with cardiovascular disease outcomes. Hs-CRP is known to be predictive of heart attacks, strokes, and diabetes. The JUPITER trial showed 1 in 12 people with an elevated hs-CRP will suffer a cardiovascular event in four years. 1 in 20 with high hs-CRP will die.[173] We need to find the cause of elevated hs-CRP and get rid of it . . . fast.

Another marker of inflammation is PLA2, otherwise known as phospholipase A2. This enzyme is elevated in patients with active coronary artery disease and contributes to damage in many ways. PLA2 sits on coronary plaque and produces free radicals. It is very specific for heart inflammation. If this number is high, you can bet heart blockages are forming.[174] Elevated PLA2 is also associated with future congestive heart failure.[175] A 2014 article discussed how this enzyme actually breaks down the HDL molecules. This means PLA2 is not just a marker of disease, but actually increases risk by destroying the ever-important HDL. I routinely test my patients for PLA2, but your typical cardiologist has never even heard of it.

★LIVE WELL: Get tested for and get rid of CRP and PLA2, two bad boys for your heart.

There are many ways to reduce inflammation. Eating Paleo nutrition is the best way because you are avoiding the foods that trigger inflammation such as sugar, dairy, grain, and even caffeine. You may also consider a food sensitivity panel from companies such as ALCAT or US Biotek to specifically highlight problem foods. Avoiding chemicals and toxins will also put out the fire. Certain infections, such as H. pylori, chlamydia, and viruses may cause vascular inflammation and need to be treated naturally (not with pharmaceuticals).

I will discuss supplements in Chapter 16, but certain nutrients, such as resveratrol, turmeric, vitamins C and E, n-acetyl cysteine, and omega-3 fish oil, are just several of the many natural ways to reduce inflammation. Exercise is proven to lower CRP, but keep the duration under 1 hour, as prolonged exercise has the opposite effect.[176] Maintain good dental hygiene, avoid root canals, and floss every day, all of which reduce inflammation. Read more about the importance of dental health in Chapter 15.

OXIDATIVE STRESS AND FREE RADICALS

We see evidence of oxidation in our everyday lives. When iron in metal oxidizes, rust is the result. The browning of a cut apple or avocado is oxidation at work. The human body has a similar process. Everyone knows oxygen is one of the most critical elements in the body and is essential for life; without it, humans die in just a few minutes. But oxygen can turn deadly because when it is utilized in cellular reactions, free radicals are naturally generated. A free radical is an atom robbed of an electron, making it highly reactive and unstable, capable of setting off a chain reaction damaging membranes, tissues, and even causing cell death. The free radicals serve a purpose (as does everything the body produces) such as killing off bacterial and viral invaders. Fortunately, a healthy body generates antioxidants, which are the peacekeepers designed to combat the reckless free radicals.

★**LIVE WELL**: he human body is the best pharmacy.

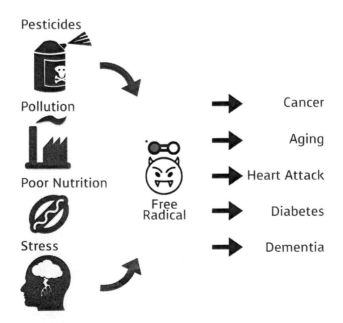

Oxidative stress is defined as a situation where the free radicals outnumber the antioxidants. This scenario is due to bad food, chemicals, and heavy metals. Elevated blood sugar causes oxidative stress. Oxidative stress is thought to be a culprit in cardiovascular disease, cancer, diabetes, dementia and Parkinson's. Even the aging process itself is thought to be an accumulation of damage from oxidative stress. If oxidative stress is too much for a cell to handle, it dies.

★**LIVE WELL**: Oxygen is essential to our bodies, but it can produce free radicals; if they outnumber our antioxidants, it can lead to oxidative stress.

Oxidation of LDL changes it and allows these particles to easily migrate through the blood vessel wall. This damaged LDL is not easily recognized by the liver and circulates longer in the blood stream. Studies find the risk of plaque is much greater in people with higher levels of oxidized LDL.[177] Oxidative stress increases platelet activity, leading to sticky blood, and also recruits cells of inflammation to the area. Some free radicals, known as reactive oxygen species, bind up nitric oxide, inhibiting the ability of a blood vessel to expand. This can lead to spasm of arteries, causing a heart attack or, at the least, symptoms of chest discomfort and shortness of breath.

Two blood tests that measure oxidative stress are lipid peroxides and myeloperoxidase. Checking levels of homocysteine also helps to determine oxidative stress burden. The more homocysteine present, the more oxidation involved. Is your doctor testing you for these markers?

We know oxidized lipids are associated with coronary disease, but recently oxidative stress has been found to be a culprit in atrial fibrillation, an irregular heart rhythm.[178] A study found vitamin C before open-heart surgery dramatically reduces post-operative atrial fibrillation. Similar results are seen with vitamin E.[179] Eight randomized trials combined to show n-acetyl cysteine (NAC- a compound with anti-oxidant properties) reduces post-operative atrial fibrillation.[180] These simple therapies are NEVER used by heart surgeons. Low levels of vitamin E are associated with decreased success of cardioversion, a procedure to restore normal rhythm from atrial fibrillation.[181] Lastly, L-arginine is an amino acid that forms the blood vessel dilator, nitric oxide. Supplementing L-arginine helps to relax the arteries, which counteracts the effects of free radical accumulation.[182] Again, these therapies are never considered by your typical M.D.

Antioxidant supplements serve to boost glutathione, the main antioxidant in the body. Eating Paleo with an abundance of animal protein will boost glutathione. Although not quite Paleo, grass-fed whey protein is an excellent supplement for this purpose, as long as you are not sensitive to whey. My preferred source of protein comes from beef in our Paleo Fuel powder. N-acetyl cysteine forms glutathione. Alpha lipoic acid, resveratrol, vitamin C, and CoQ 10 are excellent antioxidants. Vitamin E travels with LDL to prevent oxidative damage. Saturated fats are very resistant to oxidative damage, which makes them great for cooking. Polyunsaturated vegetable oils such as corn and soy are prone to oxidation. They increase disease. A trial done many years ago in the 1960's showed cooking with animal fat is superior to corn oil, and even olive oil, when it comes to life and death![183]

AUTOIMMUNE

The term autoimmune literally means the body is attacking itself. It is well known autoimmune conditions, such as lupus, rheumatoid arthritis, psoriasis, and Hashimoto's, are associated with a much higher cardiovascular risk. These patients produce high amounts of inflammation, exhibit decreased exercise ability, and take some pretty toxic pharmaceuticals. Our immune cells are critical and we cannot live without them, but when they are activated, it had better be for a good reason such as defending the body against foreign invaders. Historically, these include bacteria, viruses, and other infectious pathogens. Unfortunately, today the immune system is on high alert from other stimuli, most of it coming from unnatural foods and chemicals. The explosion of people with allergies, eczema, and asthma are excellent examples of the immune system in action.

> ★LIVE WELL: Autoimmune conditions in our population are exploding. Witness all the TV commercials for pain pills and immune-suppressing drugs.

The body has two immune divisions, innate and adaptive. The INNATE division is the first line of defense, immediately called into action when invaders are present. Cells such as neutrophils, mast cells, and macrophages are part of this army. Not only do they search and destroy, but they also "present" the foreign invaders to the ADAPTIVE immune division for long-term protection. Macrophages are found in atherosclerotic plaque. They release inflammatory mediators like IL-6 and TNF-alpha, and cause plenty of oxidative damage. These mediators also recruit smooth muscle cells to the area to strengthen the plaque. This is all part of the body's repair mechanism in response to poor nutrition and chemicals.

The adaptive system is mostly lymphocytes with a memory so you don't get the same infection twice. For example, chicken pox is a virus that leads to symptoms once in your life. The next time your body encounters that virus, the memory lymphocytes are called into action and you do not develop symptoms. Interestingly, exposure to the chicken pox virus boosts our immune system and prevents the disease known as shingles. Adults are no longer exposed to the chicken pox virus due to mass vaccination against this benign disease. Subsequently, unhealthy adults are not protected against the reactivation, commonly known as shingles. Merck is quite happy at this phenomenon and will gladly sell you a shingles shot. According to the manufacturer, the vaccine reduces the risk of shingles from 3% to 2%. Not a whopping benefit. I will take my chances with good nutrition and chemical avoidance, or travel to Amish country for re-exposure to wild chicken pox.

★LIVE WELL: Innate immune systems attack foreign invaders in our body. Adaptive systems contain a memory stick, so they avoid chicken pox the second time around.

Speaking of vaccines, is it possible the constant barrage of these immune stimulators leads to negative cardiovascular effects? I once consulted on a patient who suffered a heart attack just six hours after a flu shot. Other doctors would not see the correlation and attributed the heart attack to a chance event. There are no random events in the human body, everything happens for a reason. Medical literature contains many case reports of cardiac complications from vaccines, and the federal government's Vaccine Adverse Events Reporting System (VAERS) contains thousands of reports of vaccine induced cardiovascular injury. There are no long-term follow-up studies on side effects.

ENTER GLUTEN

Celiac disease is a dramatic immune reaction to gluten consumption, characterized by bloody bowel movements and severe gastrointestinal damage. Gluten is a small protein found in wheat, barley, and rye. It is also a common food additive. Cardiac issues are frequent in celiac patients, but often the heart can repair itself by avoiding gluten.[184] When most people eat gluten, an autoimmune cascade is set in motion as the body attacks this foreign invader. A scenario is created where the immune/invader combination is very irritating to the body. It sets up inflammation and oxidative stress as described above. The immune/invader combination can travel around the body and deposit itself in joints, arteries, the brain, etc. The immune system finds cells and body parts that look attractive and attacks them. This is how most people develop autoimmune diseases such as rheumatoid arthritis, type 1 diabetes, and hypothyroidism. That's correct, thyroid dysfunction is caused by the immune response to poor nutrition and chemicals. The immune response may not lead to symptoms, but it can cause coronary artery disease. Once again, the body forms vascular plaque as a response to injury. After millions of years of evolution, our body does not make mistakes. Other autoimmune conditions exist in cardiology such as rheumatic heart disease, pericarditis, myocarditis, and endocarditis. All of these are likely caused by an infection or chemical exposure.

LEAKY GUT SYNDROME

How do gluten, poor nutrition, chemicals, pharmaceuticals, heavy metals, pesticides, chlorine, and fluoride lead to inflammation, oxidation, and immune stimulation? By causing a leaky gut. Leaky Gut Syndrome is a newly recognized condition your average medical practitioner is unlikely to know about. This diagnosis was not discussed in my medical school, residency, or fellowship. In 2014, leaky gut, also known as increased intestinal permeability, is finally getting the attention it deserves. Search intestinal permeability in pubmed.gov and you will find over 10,000 articles.

Do you have a leaky gut?

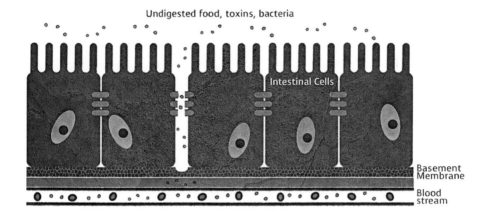

The gut lining is damaged from poor nutrition and chemicals, and becomes very porous, thus allowing undigested food particles and bacteria to get into the blood stream. The human immune system recognizes these as foreign invaders, igniting a massive inflammatory and autoimmune response. I believe a leaky gut leads to Leaky Heart Syndrome. The endothelium lines blood vessels. When leaky, the endothelium no longer functions to keep damaged LDL and other inflammatory stimulators out of the vessel wall. Coronary artery blockage is the end result.

In any person with symptoms or signs of disease, assume a leaky gut. Cyrex Labs in Phoenix performs an intestinal permeability panel. This blood test checks for bacteria particles and antibodies, to the two proteins that manage the junction between cells lining the intestines, zonulin and occludin. If antibodies are present, the gut is leaking and allowing unwanted food particles, bacteria, and other pathogens into the body.

CASE STUDY

Emily G. came to see me when she was pregnant because her blood pressure was a little high. Talking with Emily during her initial visit, she also admitted to frequent muscle aches and joint pains. It took her a while to get going in the morning. Blood testing revealed mild elevation in her markers of inflammation, and the presence of thyroid antibodies. She admitted to her love affair with bread and pasta. From there, I ordered a food sensitivity panel, which uncovered an issue with wheat, gluten, and garlic of all things.

Emily gave up the wheat and all gluten-containing foods for three weeks. On a repeat visit, she reported a 90% improvement in muscle and joint pains. Maybe more importantly, her blood pressure was in the normal range, and she had an uneventful pregnancy, successful homebirth, and beautiful baby girl.

ACTION PLAN

1. Poor nutrition and chemicals activate inflammation, oxidation, and the immune system.
2. Free radicals can lead to plenty of damage to your body
3. Get tested and make sure you know your numbers
4. Find the cause of abnormal test results
5. Go Paleo, eat organic, and avoid chemicals. Watch as your abnormal blood test return to normal.

Chapter 11

GO TO SLEEP

"A good laugh and a long sleep are the two best cures for anything."
—Irish Proverb

We spend all our lives worrying about what is going on while we are awake, yet most people do not realize the importance of sleep. An estimated 60 million Americans suffer from sleep disorders or sleep deprivation. Sleep is the time when our body repairs from the mental and physical stress of the day. Hormones are secreted, lipids are formed, and proteins are synthesized during the bedtime hours. For millions of years, humans went to sleep at sundown and awoke at sunrise. There was no switch to turn on artificial lights. All animals need to sleep. We would be wise to follow the footsteps of our ancestors.

A 2013 study reported there are over 2,000 genes that work differently whether we are awake or asleep.[185] Areas of DNA code for muscle repair and memory are active at night while other segments of DNA, such as adrenal hormones, are at work in the daytime. Our body functions in a totally different manner during sleep and awake time. Cells divide, tissues repair, and growth hormones are released during sleep. Sadly, the average time most Americans go to sleep is near midnight.

According to recent studies, a good night's sleep improves learning. Whether it's a new language, how to play the guitar, or how to perfect your golf swing, sleep helps enhance your learning and problem-solving skills. Sleep also helps you pay attention, make decisions, and be creative. Get adequate sleep to become a better spouse, parent, grandparent, child, boss, or employee.

★LIVE WELL: A good night's sleep is the proper counterpart to an active life—both are necessary for good heart health.

An interesting study looked at sleep and cardiovascular events such as heart attack and stroke. During 10-15 years of follow-up, short sleepers (less than 6 hours) had a 23% higher risk of coronary artery disease compared to normal sleepers (more than 7 hours) after adjustment for all other possible factors. Short sleepers with poor sleep quality had a 79% higher risk of heart disease when compared to normal sleepers with good sleep quality. On a side note, sleeping longer than 9 hours provided no benefit.[186] Data from 1964 found those people who slept 7-8 hours had the lowest chance of dying over a 3-year follow-up.

Scientists have known for years that heart attacks are more frequent in the morning hours. The blaring alarm clock and stress of the day ahead tip some people over the edge into an unstable heart situation. But this next problem is very easy to change. The practice known as Daylight Savings Time is totally useless in this modern age and interferes with our circadian rhythm. It is not normal to change our sleep cycle by following this antiquated practice. A 2013 study identified men are at a 70% increased risk of having a heart attack on the day after the time change and 20% more likely in the first week. This is extraordinary. Considering recent presidents Bush, Clinton, Bush, LBJ, and Eisenhower all had cardiovascular disease, maybe the current president should look into abandoning Daylight Savings Time? It may save his life.[187]

★**LIVE WELL**: Get 8-9 hours of sleep each night to avoid morning heart attacks!

Add hypertension to the list of bad outcomes from a lack of sleep. Yes, not getting your Z's can lead to high blood pressure. Practicing for years as a typical cardiologist, I was frustrated by seeing patients on five anti-hypertensive drugs, yet their blood pressure was not controlled. Not once did it ever cross my mind poor sleep could be a factor. I certainly never counseled a patient regarding the need for sleep. I was only getting 5-6 hours per night and envied other doctors who could get away with less. Now I pity those doctors leading the sleep-deprived lifestyle. Anyway, back to hypertension.

A study in 2006 demonstrated poor sleep doubled the risk of hypertension. This study even corrected for other factors such as the fact poor sleepers may be more stressed, or are likely to be smokers. A similar article from 2013 found middle-age nurses had a higher risk of hypertension when they had poor sleep patterns.[188] In early 2014, a story about how poor sleep increases the risk of stroke in women made front-page news. In fact, for young women, the risk of a stroke was 8x higher in those admitting to five hours of sleep or less. The study found 10% of women age 65 and older had a stroke within four years if they had poor sleep. Another study found women who frequently feel drowsy during the daytime are at 58 percent higher risk for heart disease compared to those who rarely or never experience this symptom.[189]

Poor sleep is also associated with elevated markers of inflammation, such as CRP, TNF-alpha, fibrinogen, and interleukins. As we discussed, inflammation is caused by all the unhealthy things in our lives, from nutrition and chemicals to poor sleep. The more inflammation, the higher the risk of heart disease.[190] This is major news, and is a call to action for women to get more sleep.

★**LIVE WELL**: Get 8 hours of sleep each night to normalize blood pressure and inflammation.

Struggling to lose a few pounds? Poor sleep could be your problem. Recent studies suggest an association between sleep duration and weight gain. Sleeping less than five hours, or more than nine hours per night, appears to increase the likelihood of weight gain. In one study, recurrent sleep deprivation in men increased their preferences for high-calorie foods and their overall calorie intake. In another study, women who slept less than six hours a night were more likely to gain 11 pounds (5 kg) compared with women who slept seven hours a night. One explanation may be sleep duration affects the hormones regulating hunger—ghrelin and leptin—and stimulates the appetite. Another contributing factor may be lack of sleep leads to fatigue and results in less physical activity. Obviously, the longer you are awake, the more time there is to eat.[191]

> ★LIVE WELL: Get 8-9 hours of sleep each night to feel alert and lose weight!

POOR SLEEP IS ALSO ASSOCIATED WITH:
1. Memory loss and Alzheimer's.[192]
2. Decreased immune system function.[193]
3. Anxiety and irritability.
4. Dying younger. One study found that women with short sleep duration and poor sleep quality had over 3x the risk of dying as those who slept over 7 hours.[194]

The cause(s) of sleep problems needs to be addressed. They might be physical, mental, or both. Even counting grass-fed sheep is not going to work if you are in a bad relationship or having issues at work. Foods not on the Paleo plan negatively effect sleep quality. It doesn't matter what time you drank your coffee. The caffeine effect can last over 24 hours. Waking up in the middle of the night may be because your blood sugar is dropping and your body is craving more food, usually junk food.

ACTION PLAN: TWENTY WAYS TO A BETTER NIGHT SLEEP
1. Go to sleep just after sundown and wake at sunrise. Edison invented electricity 125 years ago. Our bodies will never adapt to it.

2. Get the electronics out of your bedroom. Cell phones, cordless phones, Wi-Fi, and computers produce electromagnetic fields. Pay attention to electronics on the other side of the headboard wall. Remove smart meters.

3. Do not watch TV in bed at night. Read a book or magazine.

4. Find your cave. Turn off all lights and invest in good window coverings.

5. Keep it cool. Most people find it difficult to sleep at extremes of too hot or cold.

6. Go Paleo and lose weight. Obese people are more prone to sleep apnea, a condition associated with cardiovascular and mental problems.

7. Get rid of the alarm clock. If you need to wake early, go to bed early.

8. Get an organic mattress. A synthetic foam mattress is loaded with off-gassing petrochemicals, flame-retardants, and other POPs (persistent organic pollutants). These conventional mattresses harbor dust mites, a source of allergies and inflammation.

9. Use a natural laundry detergent and give up the fabric softener and dryer sheets. Your body wants to breathe air, not chemicals. The nasal, sinus, and airway congestion due to allergies from these items can inhibit your sleep. Instead buy Seventh Generation, Dr. Bronner's Sal Suds, or other ecofriendly brands.

10. Do not take pharmaceutical sleep aids. Studies show an increased risk of heart attacks, aortic dissection, and cancer.[195]

11. Shower at night. This helps to relax your body and your mind. Showering or bathing also washes the chemicals you accumulated all day off the skin.

12. Avoid caffeine. Caffeine can last in your system for up to 48 hours.

13. Avoid sugar. This is a major stimulant, so get rid of the ice cream before bed.

14. Breathing techniques. Check out the free app from Saagara. My patients love it.

15. Exercise. Many studies confirm exercise improves sleep. Just don't do it too close to bedtime.[196] Practice yoga and Pilates. The benefits of yoga just keep lunging in, including better sleep.[197]

16. Get the stress out. There is nothing you can do about life's problems while in bed. You cannot cope with stress if you are sleep deprived.

17. Get sunshine. This helps to set your internal sleep clock.

18. Just say no to alcohol. It is a major inhibitor of quality sleep. Passing out drunk does not count.

19. Sleep alone. If your partner snores or tosses and turns all night, something has to give, likely your health.

20. Take natural supplements. See below.

NATURAL SLEEP SUPPLEMENTS

1. **Magnesium**

   Several studies show magnesium can improve sleep quality and reduce nocturnal awakenings. Along with contributing to a good night's sleep, this nutrient helps to maintain normal muscle and nerve function, keeps heart rhythm steady, supports a healthy immune system, and keeps bones strong.

2. **Melatonin**

   A hormone that regulates the normal sleep/wake cycle, melatonin is useful as an occasional sleep aid, and is especially effective against jet lag. According to research, the body naturally produces melatonin after the sun goes down, letting us know it's time to fall asleep. Supplemental melatonin assists with this process. Cherries appear to boost melatonin. Take 60-90 minutes before sleep.

3. **L-theanine**

   An amino-acid derivative found in green tea, theanine is known to trigger release in the brain of GABA, a calming neurotransmitter, which promotes relaxation and reduces anxiety. Unfortunately, the body has difficulty absorbing GABA, which is the reason experts recommend theanine. This is easily absorbed and boosts levels of GABA. Avoid green tea after 3 pm.

4. **Valerian**

   Many experts recommended this herb to reduce the amount of time it takes to nod off. According to the NIH, valerian has sedative properties, and it may increase the amount of GABA.

5. **5-HTP**

   A compound derived from the amino acid L-tryptophan, 5-HTP acts as a precursor to serotonin, which is a neurotransmitter essential for a good night's sleep. A small 2009 study of eighteen people found those who took a product containing 5-HTP needed less time to fall asleep, slept longer, and reported improved sleep quality.

6. **Lavender**

   Aromatherapy with a couple sprays of lavender oil has many proponents. Several patients of mine are fans of this herb.

7. **Chamomile Tea**

   Most people find any herbal tea to be soothing at bedtime, but chamomile is known to work very well.

8. **Lemon Balm**

   In one study of people with minor sleep problems, 81% of those who took an herbal combination of valerian and lemon balm reported sleeping much better than those who took a placebo.

9. **Phenibut (β-Phenyl-γ-aminobutyric acid)**

   Phenibut is similar to GABA, but easily crosses the blood-brain barrier, allowing for better efficacy. This is a prescription drug in Russia. Phenibut should be used under the guidance of a physician, as it can be addictive.

10. **B vitamins**

    B12 as methylcobalamin and folate (B9) as methylfolate are critical for neurotransmitter formation (and many other functions). The vast majority of vitamins contain the cheap forms of B12 as cyanocobalamin and folate as folic acid. These synthetic variants do not work well in our bodies, given 50% of the population contain a genetic defect in methylation. Make sure you know your methylation genetics. Check with your natural doctor for dosing on B vitamins.

Your best bet is to speak with a natural doctor and see what supplements are right for you. If you are reading this book in the middle of the night, shut it and go to sleep.

Chapter 12

GET OFF YOUR BUTT

"Just Do It, Then Do It Again"
—Nike Slogan

The word exercise makes a lot of people cringe. Just the thought of expending the energy and effort to work the body can raise your heart rate and blood pressure. If I say stress is bad, and exercise is stressful, then logic tells us exercise is bad. Consequently, I will use terms like "physical activity" and "Paleo lifestyle." Physical activity is defined as any bodily action using skeletal muscle over and above sitting or lying down.

It is obvious our Paleo ancestors did not hop on the treadmill for 45 minutes while reading a book or watching the TV. Paleo peoples had no choice but to be active on the hunt, to gather and walk to new areas while searching for food, safety, and shelter. From dusk 'til dawn, they carried their young along with all their possessions using only the strength of their legs, back, arms, and shoulders. Moving branches, rocks, and dirt was part of their daily life. These activities were all necessary for survival and for the survival of the tribe. Do you think it is easy picking vegetables all day, or stalking prey on a hunt? Give it a try some day.

The only choices in the days of the cavemen were healthy choices. Needless to say, activity was done outside in the sun or rain, and sometimes in the snow. It was communal and enjoyable—all the people working together for the same goal. According to my former medical students who lived among modern Paleo in the Philippines, they did enjoy the effort.

When and how we stay active is the subject of this chapter, but let me start with the why, especially regarding cardiovascular health. The evidence regarding the health benefits of physical activity is overwhelming. It plays a critical role in the prevention and the recurrence of coronary events and other cardiovascular problems such as congestive heart failure, hypertension, and arrhythmias. Many studies demonstrate that regular exercise and physical activity prevent primary and secondary cardiac events. In one prominent study, male Harvard University alumni without a history of cardiovascular disease (CVD) were followed for 16 years. There was a 39% reduction in cardiovascular morbidity and a 24% reduction in cardiovascular mortality in subjects with exercise energy expenditures of more than 2,000 kcal per week.[198] You don't need to go for an hour jog. A study from July 2014 found that as little as 5-10 minutes of jogging can reduce the risk of dying from cardiac arrest by one third![199]

★**LIVE WELL**: Regular exercise and physical activity prevent primary and secondary cardiac events.

Once a person is diagnosed with coronary disease, exertion training can clearly improve outcomes, and reduce their overall mortality by decreasing their risk of sudden death. Oldridge et al. performed a meta-analysis of ten trials on the effects of cardiac rehabilitation after myocardial infarction (MI). There was a 25% reduction in cardiovascular deaths among rehabilitation patients compared with controls.[200]

I believe one of the major benefits of cardiac rehab is the fact that patients get to work out with other people who carry a similar diagnosis. There is comfort in sharing stories of recovery. The mental is just as important as the physical. This is especially true for people who would otherwise be socially isolated.

★**LIVE WELL**: Cardio training and rehabilitation are proven to benefit those suffering from coronary disease.

The benefits of physical activity on the heart and vascular system may result from an improvement in risk factors, such as reducing blood pressure, improving lipids, and lowering blood sugar. Endothelial function improves, which enhances blood flow, and blood-clotting activity reaches a healthy state.[201] Physical activity improves markers of congestive heart failure, heart function, and is associated with improved markers of blood viscosity, otherwise known as stickiness.[202] The more sluggish the blood flow, the higher the risk of damage to blood vessels. A similar study was done on obese women and found exercise decreased clotting activity. Finally, physical exertion lowers markers of inflammation, therefore lowering heart disease risk.

It is obviously in every individual's interest to assume the responsibility for their own health and embrace physical activity as an extremely effective, safe, and inexpensive way to lower cardiac risk. But I am the first to admit this is not easy. The world is against us. We are all under work and family stress, which pull us in other directions. Every second I am spending writing this book is time I could be improving my own health. Oh, the sacrifices I make to change the world! The bottom line is you MUST make the time to walk, swim, jog, bike, hike, and increase muscle strength. Use it or lose it. Don't wait too long. The older we get, the more difficult it is to build muscle.

★**LIVE WELL**: Regular exercise is a necessity for good heart health, not an option.

There is a lot of confusion about the best forms of physical activity. Are jogging and cycling, two endeavors commonly thought of as "cardio," better than muscle-building activities? Opinions vary, but the most important thing is to do some something. The first couple weeks are the most difficult, but once you getting rolling, you can't stop. People should be exerting themselves most days of the week, but be careful—exercise can be addictive and too much exercise for too long can be dangerous and unhealthy.

There are two categories of physical activity: Cardio and Resistance. Cardio includes walking, jogging, hiking, cycling, swimming, and many other forms of aerobic activity. Resistance training builds muscle, whether using weights or your own body weight. Of course, there is considerable overlap, as doing 100 push-ups will work your muscles and your heart. Yoga is often considered a static activity yet the heart rate during this practice can rise to over 120 beats per minute.

My personal routine is to perform 20 minutes of weight training daily along with 20 minutes of cardio activity. An example would be a chest and triceps workout on Mondays followed by an outdoor hike. Tuesdays are back and biceps with sprints. Wednesdays are legs followed by outdoor or stationary bike. Thursdays are abdominals along with a light run. Friday is shoulder day followed by the bike. The weekends are reserved for family hikes, walks, bike rides, and swimming when the season is right. When the weather is right I try to bike outside, but unfortunately outdoor cycling is dangerous.

Staying active and exerting yourself should be fun; a time to get away from all the stress of life. You should look forward to your workout, knowing you are gravitating toward a healthier body, mentally and physically. Do activities you enjoy. To me, there is nothing better than a hike through the mountains with my family. Kayaking and water sports are excellent options for those near water. Take lessons so you are comfortable and are taught the correct technique.

★LIVE WELL: Regular exercise is best done outside and through activities you enjoy.

You do not need to join a gym or buy fancy equipment, so consider this money saved to pay for organic nutrition and supplements. Use your own body weight for exercises such as push-ups, pull-ups, squats, and lunges. Add dumbbells to build muscle mass or find items around the house, such as gallon jugs of water or stacks of books. Home gym equipment is usually pretty affordable.

Getting outdoors as often as possible is key. I used to run all through downtown Chicago in the middle of winter. Dress in layers and remove as needed. The fresh outdoor air and ever-changing scenery is tremendous for your mind and body. Start slow. Just because you played football 30 years ago does not qualify you as an athlete today. Many incidents of sudden death occur while exercising, but this is usually when people attempt to do too much, too fast. The bottom line is: do not climb a mountain when your main exercise for the last 25 years has been walking to the refrigerator. When in doubt, get a treadmill stress test prior to starting an exercise regimen. Having a routine physical with a doctor who will listen to your heart and check an ECG is a good idea.

You can get too much of a good thing. There is mounting evidence that marathon runners actually build more coronary artery disease than non-runners. Studies show heavy endurance activity increases markers of inflammation. Prolonged exercise may also increase the risk of heart rhythm disorders such as slow heart rates known as bradycardia, atrial fibrillation, and ventricular tachycardia.[203] In summary, exercise appears to be a J-shaped curve. Those who are the least active are at the highest risk of heart disease, but those who overdo it are also at an increased risk. Hit the sweet spot.

★LIVE WELL: Exercise is best done routinely and in moderation, not with extreme exertion.

YOGA

Although yoga has been around for many years, it seems more and more people are jumping on the band-wagon. In fact, the origin of yoga dates back thousands of years. There are many different forms and styles, so find what works for you based on comfort and location. I encourage you to try a variety before you settle on a particular brand.

The three main aims of yoga—exercise, breathing, and meditation—make it beneficial to those suffering from heart disease or those looking to prevent it. A 2014 review examined the effects of yoga on cardiovascular disease risk-factors. Their findings were nothing less than astounding. Systolic blood pressure improved, as did diastolic pressure. Heart rate was reduced as was breathing rate. Weight loss was profound. Interestingly, total cholesterol, HDL, VLDL, and triglycerides markedly improved. Lastly, diabetes markers, such as Hgb A1C and insulin resistance, moved in a positive direction.[204] In 2011, another study reported yoga decreased the occurrence of atrial fibrillation, lowered anxiety and depression, and improved the quality of life in those patients with atrial fibrillation.[205]

A program using yoga found those who followed the protocol missed 8.5 fewer days from work each year.[206] In a separate study, a research group from the Boston University School of Medicine tested yoga's effects on lower back pain. Over twelve weeks, one group of volunteers practiced yoga while the control group continued with standard treatment for back pain. The reported pain for yoga participants decreased by one-third, while the standard treatment group had only a five percent drop. Yoga participants also had a drop of 80% in pain medication use.[207]

★LIVE WELL: Exercise, breathing, and meditation make yoga beneficial to improving anyone's heart health.

Although for many years I recommended my patients perform yoga, sadly, I had not tried it myself. A friend of mine who is a cardiologist in Michigan had encouraged me to give it a shot, as he performs an in-office class with his patients. So finally I gave it a try, and now I am hooked. I decided on a hot yoga style. The hot yoga causes an intense sweat response, which is a great detoxification of chemicals. The heat also allows for improved stretching and flexibility, and has improved my balance and muscle tone. Remember to load up on your minerals after sweating, as they are lost through the skin. Try to find a yoga studio that uses natural cleaning products.

A quick word on clothing. I am not going to tell you what to wear. Frankly, I don't care if you work out naked. What I do care about is how you smell. One of my pet peeves is running on a beautiful trail and passing someone who smells of perfume/cologne, laundry detergent, fabric softener, or dryer sheets. Here I am, trying to stay healthy in the great outdoors, and having to breathe poison. Even worse is exercising indoors next to someone with a chemical smell. This is not good for your health. All fitness clubs and gyms douse their equipment with chemicals.

Do us both a favor. Do not use any scented products unless they are natural. Activity usually means sweat and your glands are open, ready to absorb all of the toxins. If you know people who use chemicals, tell them to stop! We cannot change the world unless we say something.

★**LIVE WELL**: Whether yoga or any other form of exercise, avoid chemicals and other artificial poisons—stay natural.

ACTION PLAN: HOW TO STAY PHYSICALLY ACTIVE

1. Do it outside as much as possible. Even in cold weather, bundle up and go. I used to ride with a cycling group in the west suburbs of Chicago. The owner's motto was, "There is no such thing as bad weather, only bad clothes." We rode in the snow countless times. When it's hot, go in the morning or late evening. Join a group or go with a partner if safety is an issue. Get sunshine.

2. Walk, hike, bike, jog, sprint, swim, kayak, stand-up paddleboard, climb, etc.

3. The best way to health is with burst activity. Burst means go hard for a while then slow or rest. Repeat. Repeat. Repeat. This would be the most Paleo-esque. Our ancestors were not running marathons.

4. Build muscle mass. Do push-ups, pull-ups, planks, squats, lunges, handstands, etc. This does not require fancy equipment or an expensive gym membership. Muscle building has been shown to lower inflammation, raise levels of testosterone, increase fat burning, lower blood glucose, and lower cardiovascular risk. Paleo people did the same all day long by lifting rocks, logs, food, and babies. You may need to purchase weights at some point to really build muscle and progress in health. Burst activity to muscle building ratio should be 1:1 as far as time goes. A great workout only takes 20-30 minutes by following this plan. Find time to do it.

5. Start slow. I know you were a star athlete in high school, but guess what? You are not in high school. For many reading this book, high school was 30-40 years ago or more. You get the point. Ease into a regular workout routine and gradually make it more rigorous.

6. Listen to the "earth music." When you are outside, listen to the birds, the trees, the wind. You will be in touch with nature. Avoiding the music distraction allows you to focus on your breathing, your position, and is much likely safer. Once in a while, it's okay to listen to your favorite songs, but try to minimize EMF exposure.

7. Walk or ride a bike instead of driving.

8. Stand instead of sitting. Get a standing desk. Stand and read. Stand while on the phone.

9. Live barefoot (as much as possible). Our ancestors did it full time. No other animal wears shoes. If you wear shoes, wear thin soles. Incorporate the concept of "Earthing" popularized by Clint Ober.

Chapter 13

HEALTHY BEVERAGES

"You will know the importance of water when it's gone."
—Unknown

N
ow that you know what to eat, let's look at what to drink. Humans can live for weeks without food, but only a few days without liquids. Our body is made of mostly water, a virtual ocean in which all life-giving activity takes place. In all beverages—whether milk, wine, coffee, or soda—water is the main ingredient. No water means no life.

The body has multiple ways to dispose of waste and toxins. None is more important than through the kidneys, a bean-shaped organ located on both sides of your lower spine. Staying well hydrated ensures there is plenty of blood flow to the kidneys to get rid of waste as urine. Also, the more fluid you drink, the less likely you are to develop constipation. Rotting food in your colon is a sure-fire way to disease. Daily bowel movements prevent this major source of toxicity. The waste of the body must get out of the body.

Fluid intake promotes health in other ways. When you are hydrated, you are able to sweat easily. Sweating is an additional path to get out toxins such as heavy metals. When your lungs produce phlegm, it carries out waste products. Hydration is also the key to mucous secretion. Proper hydration ensures stomach acid production to allow for digestion of your food. The small intestine also secretes fluid to allow easy passage of waste. If you are dehydrated, none of these important processes occur.

★**LIVE WELL**: No water, no life—plenty of water equals good heart, lung, and kidney health.

When it comes to beverages, obviously there are many choices. From coffee and tea to soda and alcohol, we need to understand the pros and cons of each option. Certainly, nothing is more critical than crystal clear water. Our Paleo ancestors drank plain agua, nothing else. They were lucky to have clean water with all the right minerals. Despite all the health claims of certain beverage makers (one product named after a reptile comes to mind), water is our number one source of hydration and the cleansing of the body.

THE IMPORTANCE OF WATER

Water makes up 75% of the human body and is necessary to sustain life. The older we get, the more water we need, as our billions of cells struggle to hold on to fluid. Think of babies and children with thick, tight skin versus the loose skin of senior citizens. A major factor in this issue is the loss of water. An excellent book on this subject is *Your Body's Many Cries for Water*. The medical doctor who wrote this book, F. Batmanghelidj, M.D., warns us to not wait for symptoms of thirst and a dry mouth. By that point, it is too late. You are already dehydrated. Older folks may not exhibit any symptoms or triggers prompting them to drink. Trust me, for sixteen years I saw many seniors come into the hospital in kidney failure because of dehydration. Summer heat waves are a well-known cause of many casualties to the elderly.

Did you know water intake is critical for heart health? High blood pressure is likely another sign of dehydration. When the body is deficient in water, blood volume is decreased, and mechanisms are set into action to maintain blood pressure. Hormones are released from the kidneys and sodium is retained. The blood vessels literally clamp down. The solution is either to drink more water or take pharmaceuticals. What is your choice? Many patients are able to stop pharmaceuticals when they improve their water intake. There is data demonstrating mineral water lowers blood pressure in people with hypertension.[208] Increasing water intake may help clear excess lipid particles.[209]

★**LIVE WELL**: Stay hydrated—dehydration leads to poor skin, high blood pressure, and kidney failure.

Do you or anyone you know swallow pharmaceuticals for heartburn? That is actually a silly question because millions of people consume these drugs for the newly labeled disease gastro-esophageal reflux disorder (GERD). Contrary to popular belief, heartburn is not from too much stomach acid, but rather it is from too little! Unfortunately, just one drop of acid in the wrong direction will cause horrible symptoms such as pain, gas, and bloating. When we are deficient in stomach acid, we do not digest our food properly. This leads to dysfunction of the lower esophageal sphincter, the muscle that controls stomach contents from going backwards. There are many ways to improve digestion, including apple cider vinegar, digestive enzymes, and acid supplements, but none of these methods are more important than water. If you are dehydrated, every part of your body is dehydrated, including your stomach. Water is critical for stomach acid and enzyme production. Now you know the cure for reflux.

★**LIVE WELL**: Try not to drink much during meals, as liquids dilute the digestive enzymes of the stomach.

Now that we know water is healthy and we should drink plenty of it, the type is certainly up for debate. The idea of paying for water would seem ridiculous to our grandparents. But if you want quality today, you must to pay for it. Most people realize municipal or city water is substandard and loaded with metals, chemical, hormones, and pharmaceuticals. In my opinion, the most important factor when it comes to water is that it does not contain the above-mentioned contaminants. Find the cleanest water possible.

Many authorities claim the energy of water is lost through processing when minerals are removed, leading to "dead" water. I can understand this viewpoint since our Paleo ancestors drank from mountain streams or fresh spring water. Reverse osmosis (RO) is criticized because all of the minerals are removed and it is often considered acidic. But the beauty of RO is that it's completely void of chemicals. Just give me plain H20 and I will get my minerals and nutrients from food and supplements. I think RO is a cost-effective option, especially for rinsing vegetables and cooking food.

If you ask me (which you are because you are reading my book), the best water is spring water. From deep in the earth, this source is clean, "alive," and full of trace minerals. My personal choice is to buy spring water in glass bottles whenever possible. Mountain Valley Spring Water and Evian are good options. You can get 5 gallon glass bottles delivered to your house.

★**LIVE WELL**: The best water is spring water, full of trace minerals, and without the chemicals.

We bought a whole-house filtration system. This ensures clean drinking water and also the same quality for your bath, shower, laundry, and dishwasher. How many times have you inhaled the cloud of steam upon opening your dishwasher? This is full of chlorine, fluoride, metals, and pharmaceuticals. Do your research and find a whole-house filtration company that suits you best; look for one that has been around for years, and that will provide customer references. Please speak to other people in your area before you spend some serious coin on this option.

HOW MUCH WATER SHOULD I DRINK?

For a typical person, on a typical day, half your body weight in ounces is a good place to start. On days when it is very hot or you are exercising, increase your intake. I always carry a half-gallon glass bottle around with me. If your urine is dark, you need a lot more water. Except after taking vitamins, urine should be pale yellow in color.

THE TRUTH ABOUT BOTTLED WATER AND PLASTIC

Think bottled water is always a safe bet? Think again—not all bottled waters are as pure as you would hope. We discussed this before, but I want to reiterate that plastic bottles contain dangerous chemicals, which can get into the water. Imagine the thin plastic bottles sitting inside a semi-truck trailer as it is shipped across country. Temperatures are very high in the summer in those conditions, literally baking the plastic into food and beverage. Lastly, bottled water very often is plain tap water. Why pay for that and subject your body to garbage?

★**LIVE WELL**: Drink at least half your body weight in ounces each day, and always in a glass bottle.

One of my favorite after-dinner treats is sparkling water or club soda. This is especially nice in the summer, as it is very refreshing. Herbal tea can be added to sparkling water for flavor. My patients agree, it helps to curb a sweet tooth after meals. Just make sure to drink this at least 30 minutes after a meal so as not to dilute stomach acid and digestive enzymes. Because of the carbonation (which interferes with digestion and leads to osteoporosis), I would not recommend drinking it too often.

COFFEE

Are you reading this chapter while enjoying a cup of coffee? If you are, think twice, especially if it's not organic. Debate rages on about the health benefits and dangers of everyone's favorite pick-me-up. As you know, I grew up in Chicago and I can remember sitting across the kitchen table from my dad before he went to work. He drank coffee, so of course, I drank it too. There I was, ten years old and drinking coffee. Not a good habit to start.

The one thing I hate about coffee is the addiction. I felt horrible waking up in the morning when one of my boys wanted to play, and my response was, "Let me make some coffee first." How does that sound to a kid? I do not want my children having any addictions. Let's look at the pros and cons of java.

Coffee is brewed from the roasted or baked seeds of several species of an evergreen shrub. Coffee is grown in over 70 countries, primarily in Latin

America, South America, Southeast Asia, and Africa. Once ripe, coffee beans are picked, processed, and dried to yield the seeds inside. The seeds are then roasted to varying degrees, depending on the desired flavor, before being ground and brewed to create coffee. Coffee drinking started in the 1500's. For millions of years, we never touched the stuff.

★**LIVE WELL**: Coffee is an addiction and any addiction is bad.

One of my closest friends is the head of oncology at a major university. He knows I am anti-coffee so he sends me articles and studies espousing all the benefits of "black gold," as he calls it. There are plenty of studies extolling the virtues of your morning joe, but quite simply, it is not Paleo food. Our ancestors never drank it, and neither should we. There is a list of bad foods for your health headed by sugar, grain, corn, soy, and dairy. Coffee is somewhere on the list, and depending on the person, could rank high or low.

There is plenty of controversy regarding coffee consumption and health. A study done in 1988 showed those who consumed 10 or more cups per day had a 300% increased risk of heart attack. Don't laugh; if a cup is 8 ounces, it only takes a few large Starbucks to get to that level. In that same study, 1-2 cups per day increased risk by 40%.[210] A similar study backed up those findings.[211]

The risk of coffee and heart disease may depend on your genetics. Some people are fast metabolizers of caffeine and therefore may benefit from coffee consumption. It appears the slow metabolizers, those who do not break down caffeine well, may have an increased risk from caffeine. This is a simple blood test. Lastly, a 2013 study involving over 43,000 patients found coffee consumption of over 4 cups per day increased the risk of dying by over 50% in those aged 55 and younger.[212]

★**LIVE WELL**: Some studies found an increased risk of heart attacks in coffee drinkers.

In the first few hours after coffee is consumed, blood pressure increases. For those who drink coffee for years, on average, hypertension risk is not increased.[213]

Caffeine itself clearly raises blood pressure, but there is something about the other biologically active ingredients in coffee that likely offsets the negatives. Again, it comes back to the individual. Coffee MAY be a problem in YOU. If you are hypertensive, you should break the coffee addiction and see what it does for your blood pressure and the rest of your body.

There are many positive studies on coffee. One showed coffee improves HDL scavenger function, thus removing cholesterol from plaque.[214] Coffee also appears to decrease LDL oxidation.[215] Some evidence points to coffee reducing the risk of diabetes, gout, dementia, and Parkinson's disease. Coffee may even decrease cancer risk. The coffee bean has a multitude of antioxidants that prevent free radical damage in the body, which is likely the source of its protective effects. A final point, long term outcome trials are not randomized, where one group gets coffee and the other doesn't. Do those who drink coffee have other habits (more exercise, less sugar, less calories, smoke less) that provide benefits?

★LIVE WELL: If you have any health issues, coffee and caffeine may be the sources.

Coffee is one of the most chemically sprayed crops in the world, especially in third-world countries where chemical dangers are not recognized. According to the Environmental Protection Agency, coffee that's not organic contains residue from pesticides and chemical fertilizers, which may cause cancer, skin or eye irritation, nervous system problems, or hormone imbalance. If you are going to drink coffee, make it organic. Organic coffee, which is produced on farms by the strict standards of the U.S. Department of Agriculture (USDA), is free of chemical pesticides and fertilizers. Organic farms use fewer non-renewable sources, like petroleum, and workers aren't exposed to harmful chemicals. There aren't any chemicals leaking into nearby soil, drinking water, or carried by air. Before a farm can be certified as organic, they must apply organic practices for three years. Remember, if it kills bugs, it will kill us.

At this point, I want to mention the obvious. Billions are spent on lattés and cappuccinos every year. If you drink a $5 beverage daily, that equates to $2000 per year. Yet, so many complain about the cost of organic and grass-fed meat, while wasting money at the local coffee shop. How much money is wasted on junk food in general? Add it up yourself and you will be amazed.

When all of the data and studies are reviewed, the jury is mixed on coffee. Once again, since coffee was not available to our Paleo ancestors, we should not be drinking it. I have seen many patients with complaints from racing hearts and palpitations to anxiety and fatigue that all improved once they quit drinking coffee. I have yet to find a person who quit coffee and didn't feel better. If you suffer from any medical problems, look at everything in your life, including caffeine and coffee consumption. If you drink coffee, make it organic, don't overdo it, and skip the sugar. My choice on special occasions is organic, decaf French Roast.

> ★**LIVE WELL**: Do you suffer from palpitations or heart racing? It could be from caffeine.

BREWED TEAS: BLACK, GREEN AND HERBAL

When it comes to a beverage other than water, my personal choice is a variety of herbal teas such as dandelion, chamomile, and mint. All the warmth I remember from my childhood, none of the caffeine. And let me tell you, there is nothing better than ice-cold mint tea on a hot summer day. We use the mint from our garden. I throw it into hot water and let it sit for a few hours for the water to cool. Then I transfer it into glass jars and refrigerate. You want to drink it within 4-5 days. But with so many different kinds of teas touting various health benefits, how do you know which ones are legitimate?

A study published in the *Journal of Toxicology* examined off-the-shelf black, green, white, and oolong tea bags via toxic element testing. In all, thirty different teas were tested. All of the teas were found to contain lead, some of which had unsafe levels for pregnant and lactating women. In 20% of the brewed tea, aluminum levels were above the recommended guidelines, and in some of the black teas, manganese levels were excessive. Overall, toxic contamination was found in most of the teas and some of the teas were considered unsafe. Tea may be high in fluoride. Unfortunately, there isn't standard routine testing done on tea.[216] Even organic tea may contain metals.

A January 2014 publication looked at experimental studies in both animals and humans regarding the effects of tea. Both black and green tea benefit cardiovascular health and can reduce the risk of stroke. There's also strong evidence about the positive effects of tea on endothelial function and LDL cholesterol.[217]

★**LIVE WELL**: Drinking black or green tea is probably better than coffee, but again—make it organic.

Black Tea

There is a long list of benefits from drinking black tea. The plant is the same as green tea, only this variety is oxidized in a process that gives it a stronger flavor and more caffeine. A 2013 review found black tea reduces blood pressure, cholesterol, and markers of inflammation.[218] Numerous studies found a decreased risk of stroke in tea drinkers. A 2013 meta-analysis found a 21% lower risk of both stroke incidence and mortality from stroke among those with a high tea intake in comparison with low.[219]

Black tea has about the same amount of caffeine as coffee, so be careful if you are sensitive. I do not believe the side effects of any treatment, synthetic or natural, are likely worth any purported benefits. So if you don't feel well on any food or supplement, don't take it. Earl Grey is a type of black tea with bergamot (oil of citrus) added. This oil, derived from an orange-like fruit, has some data regarding lipid improvement and blood pressure effects.[220]

Green Tea

In a study published in *Stroke*, 82,369 Japanese participants filled out dietary questionnaires on green tea consumption frequency. The subjects were followed for an average of 13 years. In comparison with infrequent tea drinkers, two to three cups of green tea per day were associated with a 14% lower risk of stroke, and drinking more than four cups per day with a 20% reduction.[221] When consumed after eating, green tea may reduce blood pressure. Green tea lowers triglycerides and contains antioxidants, which protect heart and blood vessels.

Green tea contains caffeine but much less than black tea or coffee. If you are dealing with sleep issues, anxiety, or racing heart feelings, you may do better without green tea and beverages containing caffeine.

★**LIVE WELL**: Drinking black or green tea can reduce blood pressure, reduce risk of stroke, and increase antioxidants.

ALCOHOL CONSUMPTION: A SLIPPERY SLOPE

Let me start this paragraph off by saying alcohol is not Paleo. Our ancestors never drank beer, wine, or vodka. Along with smoking and obesity, excessive alcohol consumption is a leading cause of premature death in the United States. I know studies are often used in this book to back up an argument or make a point. Candidly, studies often show improved health in those who consume alcohol. But the question remains: are there other factors that make the alcohol drinkers healthier (more money, more exercise, eat better)?

According to a study published in the *Mayo Clinic Proceedings*, light to moderate alcohol intake is associated with a decreased risk of coronary artery disease, congestive heart failure, diabetes mellitus, stroke, and death. Light to moderate means: For women, one drink per day; for men, it is no more than two drinks per day. Once the moderate threshold is surpassed, the higher the level of alcohol intake, the higher the cardiovascular risk.[222]

The toxic effects of alcohol on the liver are well known, but cardiac issues tend to receive little publicity. Heavy alcohol use can lead to atrial fibrillation, hypertension, non-ischemic dilated cardiomyopathy, and stroke. The risk is especially high for young drinkers, who tend to drink to excess or binge drink more often than their older counterparts. For males between the ages of 15 and 59, alcohol abuse is the third leading risk factor for premature death behind smoking and obesity.[223]

★**LIVE WELL**: Studies are mixed on alcohol, but it is not Paleo and is essentially straight sugar. Beer belly is appropriately named.

Alcohol is pure sugar and my belief is that alcoholism in many cases is a sugar addition. Personally, when I am strictly Paleo, avoiding all sugars and starchy carbs, I crave alcohol. Passing by our small liquor cabinet, I long for a small shot of tequila (organic of course). Many health authorities point to the high antioxidant levels in red wine as the source of health benefits. But those same beneficial nutrients can be found in the grapes themselves or in vegetables. Doctors should never encourage patients to drink alcohol, but sometimes do so to justify their own alcoholism.

SODA

I cannot even fathom the amount of soda I drank from early childhood to the age of 34. As a kid, I would sit alongside my brother and sister as we anxiously awaited the arrival of the "Pop Man." He would drop off the sugary liquid at our doorstep and we would guzzle it down, satisfying our addiction. On my second date with Heather, I showed up with a can of diet Mountain Dew. She warned me there would be no third date if I drank that poison again.

Can you believe a single can of soda contains the equivalent of 10 teaspoons of sugar? This leads to a blood sugar spike, and an insulin dump from the pancreas. To say this is an unprecedented shock to the system is a gross understatement. Our body must react to this poison bolus in a similar way as ants when their hill is stepped on. In other words, if our cells could talk, they would say, "What the #$%& is going on?" Actually our cells do talk—it's called heart disease and cancer.

★**LIVE WELL**: One can of soda equals ten teaspoons of sugar!

Over time, studies show sugary drinks lead to diabetes and insulin resistance, not to mention weight gain and other health problems.[224] Harvard researchers recently linked soft drinks to obesity (those smart Ivy Leaguers). The study found twelve-year-olds who drank soda were more likely to be obese than those who didn't, and for each serving of soda consumed daily, the risk of obesity increased 1.6 times.[225] Sugar from soda also leads to hypertension.[226]

Soda may increase cancer risk. Pancreatic cancer was higher in women who drank sodas regularly.[227] Endometrial cancer risk was also double in soda drinkers.[228] Soda contains phosphoric acid, which interferes with the body's ability to absorb calcium and can lead to osteoporosis, cavities, and bone softening. Phosphoric acid interacts with stomach acid, slowing digestion, and blocking nutrient absorption. Carbonation also leaches bone calcium. Cola lowers bone density.[229]

★**LIVE WELL**: Excessive soda drinking can lead to diabetes, obesity, hypertension, and even cancer.

Soda can lower nitric oxide in the body, which leads to vascular constriction and causes blood pressure to rise. Additionally, it is well known soda manufacturers load their drinks with plenty of salt to ensure the consumer is thirsty for more soda. Salt doesn't taste great in drinks, so sugar is added to cover up the salty taste. Magnesium is used up to metabolize sugar, therefore is not available for hundreds of other activities. This is another example where the body is trying to clear out toxins, chemicals, and bad food instead of using its resources to thrive.

Sodas contain high fructose corn syrup. Most of this corn has been genetically modified and there are no long-term studies showing the safety of GMO crops. GMO corn works by destroying the intestines of bugs. If it damages the bug's guts, what is it doing to humans? Know anyone with heartburn, gas, or bloating? Also, the process of making high fructose corn syrup involves traces of mercury, the health ramifications of which are discussed in my chapter "Heavy Metal Madness."

★**LIVE WELL**: Sodas contain high levels of fructose and phosphoric acid, which damage our intestines, stomach, and our bones.

At some point in college, I thought diet soda was a healthier option than regular cola. Along with millions of other Americans, I was horribly wrong. Diet drinks contain artificial flavors, which are likely more harmful than the sugar they replace. Aspartame, for example, is linked to many different health problems, including seizures, multiple sclerosis, brain tumors, diabetes, and emotional disorders. It converts to methanol, which breaks down to formaldehyde and formic acid. Formaldehyde is used to embalm dead bodies and causes cancer.[230] Diet sodas increase the risk of metabolic syndrome components such as low HDL, small dense LDL, and insulin resistance.[231] Diet soda does not cause weight loss. If the above studies weren't enough to reason to quit, scientists found women who drank two or more diet beverages each day were 30 percent more likely to experience a heart attack or similarly dangerous cardiovascular "event," and 50 percent more likely to die.[232]

★LIVE WELL: Soda contains artificial colorings, salt, fluoride, caffeine, and sugar substitutes, which can lead to multiple health problems, but not to weight loss!

Most sodas contain caffeine. Similar to the effects of coffee and tea, many people do not tolerate the effects of caffeine, which can include heart palpitations and high blood pressure. The water used in soda is just simple tap water and most likely contains chemicals such as chlorine, fluoride, and heavy metals. Lastly, soda causes plaque build-up on the teeth and leads to cavities and gum disease, which are associated with heart disease! Read more on dental issues and heart disease in Chapter 15.

ENERGY DRINKS

How many children must die before the beverages known as "energy drinks" are pulled from the market? It seems every day the news media is carrying word of another tragedy. These products should be illegal in the hands of children, and the public needs to know the risks of these drinks. Producers of these poisons will claim there is no definitive proof of danger, but there is not proof they are safe either. The burden of proof needs to be on the manufacturers. Google the terms "Red Bull" and "death", and over 64 million entries show up. This issue hits home, since my brother-in-law lost his brother (a heavy energy drink consumer) to a massive heart attack at the age of 39.

What makes these drinks dangerous is the high caffeine and sugar content. Some contain the caffeine equivalent of four cups of coffee, and sugar can range up to 30 grams, the same as in most candy bars. The combination of sugar and caffeine is a major problem. When people drink several of these beverages in a short period of time, it is life-threatening. You may be wondering if coffee with sugar poses a similar problem; I am sure it does.

Heart rate and blood pressure usually go up during physical activity. Energy drinks raise heart rate and blood pressure, according to a 2014 study.[233] Put exercise and energy drinks together and you create a dangerous mix. A study presented at the Radiological Society of North America meeting in 2013 found evidence of increased heart strain on cardiac MRI screenings in those consuming energy drink. The likely culprit in many cases of sudden death related to energy drinks is coronary spasm. The artery supplying blood to the heart simply collapses. Sadly, there is a startling increase in children using energy drinks.

This is big business. The Monster Energy Drink Corporation is valued at 12 billion dollars. An Austrian company owns Red Bull, the standard when it comes to energy drinks, with sales of over 5 billion cans per year. Red Bull's slogan is, "it gives you wings." You will need wings in order to get to the emergency room quickly. I am not a big believer in the government telling us what we can and cannot do. This is especially true since the government is owned by corporate America and is usually wrong when it comes to health recommendations. But we need to draw the line and say energy drinks CANNOT be consumed by minors.

★LIVE WELL: Energy drinks and exercise is a dangerous mix, increasing heart rate and heart strain.

KOMBUCHA

Attractive packaging has helped boost the kombucha trend, but this tea is far from new. It has been around for more than 2,000 years, going back to ancient China. Kombucha is made by fermenting sweet black tea with the Kombucha "mushroom." In actuality, Kombucha isn't technically a mushroom. Instead, it's a pancake-like culture of yeasts and bacteria that forms after fermentation, and which resembles a mushroom in shape and color. Given the caffeine issue, we shouldn't overdo kombucha, but it makes for a nice treat or an afternoon pick-up. Try to find a low-sugar option like the Multi-Green by GT Dave.

BREAST MILK

There are some crazy adults out there drinking human breast milk under the guise of muscle building or general health benefits. I understand human milk is very nutritious and we are built to consume it, from our newborn to toddler years. If there are web sites and organizations where one can purchase human milk, let it go to infants whose mothers could not or would not breast feed. The benefits to mother and baby are the subject of excellent books and just make common sense. The field of child psychology would need a lot less professionals if all children were breast-fed and raised by attachment parenting. In fact, we would need a lot less of all doctors, including cardiologists. But let me get back to the health benefits. For moms: less heart attacks, lower blood pressure, less diabetes, and lower risk of cancer. For babies: less future heart attacks, less cancer, less diabetes, and the list goes on and on.[234]

CASE STUDY

Michael T. is a 64 year old male with a history of hypertension. He was tried on several pharmaceuticals over the years but developed side effects to each one. He was not overweight and followed a low-carb diet. I knew trouble was brewing when he showed up for his consultation with a venti coffee from Starbucks. He drank two of these 20oz beverages daily. When asked about water consumption, he could not recall the last time he drank plain water. In my office, his blood pressure was over 180 systolic (top number). My plan for him included drinking 96oz of water daily and cutting back on the coffee to a 12oz cup of organic decaf in the morning. I also added a greens powder and beet root powder to his regimen. Two weeks later, Mike showed up in my office with a blood pressure of 128/82. He felt great and his energy level was up. He loved his new green/beet juice combo.

ACTION PLAN

Water is critical to health. All living things on this planet need it to survive. Their cells are bathed in it. But quality is as important as quantity. The water must be clean and free of chemicals and pollutants. Drink out of glass whenever possible. Drink a variety of waters. Coffee has plenty of supporting data, but be careful. Coffee is not Paleo, is addictive because of the caffeine, and can interfere with digestion. In many patients, the caffeine may lead to heart rhythm problems and hypertension. Opt for organic tea (preferably herbal) instead. Alcohol is another beverage with plenty of health hype, but do not be fooled. This liver toxin is not Paleo, raises blood sugar, and can cause heart damage. Finally, soda may be the biggest poison in society and is certainly detrimental to our health and that of our children. The sugar, the carbonation, the artificial ingredients, and the aluminum can all add up to disaster. Break the habit.

Drink:

1. Clean water
2. Herbal tea
3. Green tea or black tea
4. Kombucha
5. Club soda or sparking water

Limit:

1. Coffee
2. Alcohol

Avoid:

1. Dairy
2. Soda
3. Diet soda
4. Energy drinks

Chapter 14

THE WONDERS OF CHIROPRACTIC CARE

"Medicine is the study of disease and what causes man to die.
Chiropractic is the study of health and what causes man to live."
—**B. J. Palmer**, son of the founder of chiropractic, D. D. Palmer

T he most incredible event happened on the night of our wedding. Actually, many events from the night stand out, but I want to share a particularly amazing story. My wife's grandfather attended our wedding, and during the cocktail hour, he passed out. Grandpa David was breathing, but his pulse was slow and thready. As he lay on the ground, Heather bent down, in her wedding dress, and gave him a cervical chiropractic adjustment! Within a few seconds, he was awake and alert. Shortly thereafter he was walking around and able to enjoy the rest of the wedding. The room was full of my cardiology partners (who could do nothing) and a beautiful woman in white saved the evening.

Grandpa suffered from a common faint, sometimes called vasovagal syncope. I saw thousands of patients with this condition, and performed thousands of tilt table tests to help with the diagnosis. NEVER had I seen a person recover as fast as Grandpa David did. I was a believer before, but that night I became completely convinced in the miracle of chiropractic after seeing my wife in action.

This chapter is not just a short homage to my wife and an attempt to earn brownie points. I have witnessed the wonders of chiropractic care hundreds of times. Children are carried into our office (and sometimes our house) listless from an ear infection and high fever. Miraculously, they are up running around within minutes after an adjustment from Heather. You name the disease, chiropractic care has a role, as the nervous system controls every cell in the body. Nerves travel from the brain through the spine and out to every organ, muscle, and even fatty tissue. If the bones of the spine are not aligned, symptoms and disease occur. If you have ever fallen out of bed, been in a car accident, or played sports, be assured your spine is misaligned and you suffer from subluxations (bones out of place). In fact, poor nutrition, chemicals, and mental stress cause plenty of damage that requires chiropractic care.

★**LIVE WELL**: No matter what the disease, chiropractic care can help.

Chiropractors have an inside joke my wife was willing to share with me. Their title, abbreviated D.C., not only stands for Doctor of Chiropractic, but also for Doctor of Cause. If the thyroid is not functioning, we should seek out the cause. Synthetic thyroid hormone replacement is not the answer, but rather is a cover -up of the problem. The thyroid is innervated by nerves that control function. If a subluxation is present in the spine where the thyroid is controlled, dysfunction begins. Most people believe chiropractic is a musculoskeletal profession. Let me state categorically that chiropractic is not about moving bones or bone on nerve conditions. In reality, it is a neurological profession that uses the musculoskeletal system to make neurological changes. Every chiropractic adjustment has a profound effect on the human body.

★**LIVE WELL**: Chiropractic care does not just re-align bones, it also makes important neurological changes.

All doctors should be doctors of cause. We have to determine the reason a person is sick. My new patient evaluation is 60 minutes long for a reason (sometimes I take longer). Doctors need time to gather information about you. This cannot be done in 15 minutes. You, the patient, have 20, 50, 80 years of history on this planet! For example, thyroid disease is not because your body lacks synthetic thyroid hormone, as there is a reason the gland is not working. Look at the following list and tell me how these issues can be discussed in a short office visit.

Thyroid dysfunction could be from:

1. A vertebral subluxation
2. Lack of iodine
3. Excess chlorine, fluoride, or bromine
4. Vitamin and mineral deficiency
5. Autoimmune attack from leaky gut, poor nutrition, and chemicals
6. Heavy metals
7. Chemical interference
8. Adrenal dysfunction
9. Stress
10. Lack of sleep

Children do not get ear infections because the eardrum lacks a surgically inserted drainage tube. All the child needed was a chiropractic adjustment and to follow Paleo nutrition. I can't even count how many children my wife has saved from this worthless and dangerous procedure, which requires Inhaled gas anesthesia. Sadly, there are reports of children having this procedure done 4-5 times.

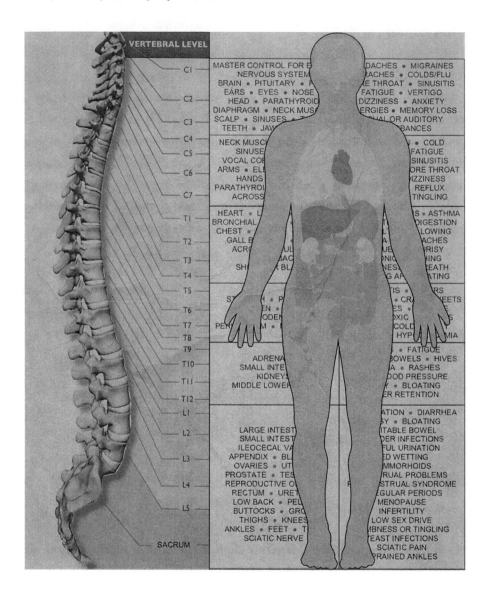

Millions of children have their tonsils removed yearly. This is part of their immune system. It is not the cause of the problem, but the result of one. The tonsils can heal if you remove the poison. Same with the adenoids. Antibiotics are rarely necessary. Seek out chiropractic care immediately. There are even board-certified chiropractic internists. They will have infinitely more knowledge on how to heal a child compared to the standard pediatrician.

Can chiropractic care help prevent and treat cardiovascular disease? Absolutely. You see, the heart and blood vessels are connected to the brain and spinal cord through millions of tiny connections. The heart is controlled by the vagus nerve and the autonomic nervous system. These nerves control heart rate, contractility, and blood pressure. If the neurologic control of the heart is dysfunctional, rhythm problems like atrial fibrillation and extra heartbeats such as PVC's will occur. In fact, you can see from the chart above that the autonomic nervous system (ANS) runs up and down the spine controlling every organ and bodily function. "Fight or flight" is the sympathetic branch, and the parasympathetic branch exerts control over things like bowel and bladder activity.

★**LIVE WELL**: Chiropractic care can help prevent and treat heart disease.

The delicate balance between the two branches of the ANS is of critical importance to cardiovascular and total body health. If one branch is dominant, because of poor nutrition, chemicals, stress, and lack of physical activity, disease will rear its ugly head. ANS balance can be determined by heart rate variability testing. The heart rate should fluctuate from beat to beat, meaning the time between beats is always changing. This is the sign of a healthy ANS and a healthy heart. People with low heart rate variability are at 5x greater risk of dying compared to those with high variability.[235]

By adjusting the 1st vertebra named the Atlas, blood pressure was lowered by 17 points, according to a study in the *Journal of Human Hypertension*. These patients were adjusted, and then followed for eight weeks in this placebo controlled trial. Ask any chiropractor and they will confirm the finding from this study. I refer most of my patients for chiropractic care not only for hypertension, but also for heart rhythm issues, heart failure, and fainting spells. In fact, I recommend every one of my patients be under the care of a chiropractor. Syncope is medical speak for passing out. This usually occurs when the brain is not communicating with the heart appropriately. Well, the pathway from the brain to the heart is through the neck. If the neck/cervical spine is misaligned, symptoms will occur. This is exactly what happened to Grandpa David.

Pain is a tremendous source of stress on the body, which undoubtedly can manifest in cardiovascular disease. Who better than the chiropractor to get you out of pain by addressing the cause? In addition, all of the over-the-counter products for pain, such as acetaminophen and ibuprofen-like drugs, are toxic and increase cardiovascular risk, not to mention liver and kidney damage. Chiropractic care lowers inflammation, which is great since people with inflammation are at high risk of heart blockages. There are many studies demonstrating chiropractic has influence on the immune system.[236] Recall from Chapter 10 how important a healthy immune system is to preventing heart disease.

Another reason I refer out to chiropractors is the fact that chest pain is often caused by an irritated muscle or displaced rib. Most patients can be quickly assessed, and once a doctor determines the heart is not involved, curative therapy from a doctor of chiropractic is imperative. Patients do not need the "million dollar work-up;" they need a chiropractic adjustment. Can you imagine the billions of dollars that would be saved if chiropractors were on staff at major hospitals? Chest pain is one of the most common reasons a person goes to the hospital, and is the source of millions of admissions per year. Costochondritis, rib misalignment, or thoracic vertebra subluxation are all causes of chest pain and shortness of breath that will respond to chiropractic care.[237]

★**LIVE WELL**: Decrease inflammation and increase immune health through chiropractic care.

Here are just a few studies proving what millions of patients already know.

CHIROPRACTIC:
1. Lowers blood pressure.[238]
2. Improves lung function: This is proven is patients with asthma and emphysema.[239]
3. Improves autonomic tone. The autonomic nervous system controls the heart, lungs, gastrointestinal tract, kidneys, bladder, sex organs and

just about every other part of the body. We need these nerves to be functioning optimally.[240]

4. Improves heart rate variability. The more your heart rate bounces around, the longer you will live.[241]

5. Decreases blood markers of inflammation. The more inflammation, the higher the risk of cardiovascular events.[242]

6. Decreases chest pain. Millions of hospital visits can be avoided with chiropractic care.[243]

When it comes to care from any doctor, you must give them time. It's taken many years to get you in the position you are in, therefore it will take time to get you back to health. Although chiropractic care will make you feel better immediately, continue regular adjustments to stay in top form. The orthodontist doesn't put braces on for a day, they stay on for months/years with frequent tweaks to get the teeth just right. The spine and human frame are no different.

Please do not ask your medical doctor or orthopedic surgeon if chiropractic is right for you. They think chiropractors and all natural doctors are "quacks." In truth, THE MEDICAL DOCTORS ARE THE QUACKS! Doctors of chiropractic are competition for those who recommend pills and procedures. Instead, ask the millions of people who see chiropractors every day. A series of chiropractic adjustments seems like a better approach than spinal surgery or short term fixes like epidural injections. Don't you agree?

★**LIVE WELL**: It may take several years to get your body back in its proper shape, but it will be worth it.

CASE STUDY

Shelley Ann is a patient of mine with recurrent syncope. Plagued by fainting episodes for years, one time she collapsed and fell into a bonfire! Luckily, the burns were not too bad and her face was spared. I performed a tilt table test that caused her to faint after her heart rate and blood pressure both dropped precipitously. The average cardiologist would put her on pills and may even suggest a pacemaker. Instead of pharmaceuticals, I gave her some recommendations. Number 1, see a chiropractor. Number 2, avoid chemicals, toxins, and electronics as much as possible. Number 3, go Paleo.

It has been several years since our initial visit, and Shelley Ann has never passed out again. She went from several episodes per year to zero. Not bad for a natural cardiology plan. Once again, every patient needs a chiropractor. If you care about your health, chiropractic is not an option, it is an absolute necessity. Don't wait for symptoms, prevent problems from starting. This is true for you, your children, and your grandchildren. Get adjusted today.

ACTION PLAN

1. Every single cell in the body is connected to the nervous system.
2. Routine daily activities can wreak havoc on your spine.
3. Chiropractic care restores health and function to your brain, nerves, and entire body.
4. Every cardiovascular problem can be improved with chiropractic care.

Chapter 15

TEETH ARE MORE THAN
A BEAUTIFUL SMILE

"Your Mouth is the Doorway to Health."
—The Drs. Wolfson

P atients often ask me if problems with their teeth and gums can lead to heart problems. The jury is in and multiple studies show that people with poor oral health are at much higher risk of cardiovascular disease.[244] Do dental problems directly cause heart disease or are the factors leading to heart disease the same as those leading to dental problems? The answer is, poor nutrition and chemicals lead to dental issues and, of course, lead to heart disease. But we also learned in Chapter 10 that infection and inflammation directly cause heart damage. So if your teeth are a source of these toxins, heart disease will follow. We all know eating sugar and carbs increases your risk of tooth decay. The sugar feeds bacteria in the mouth, which break down the strength of your teeth leading to cavities and root infections. The mouth infection leads to an inflammatory response. Inflammatory particles and immune cells in the blood lead to inflammation and damage in your heart.[245] An article from 2010 found poor oral hygiene was associated with several inflammation markers, which are also high in patients with heart disease![246]

According to Weston A. Price, the dentist who travelled the world in the 1920's, our teeth should be perfect. Not artificial movie star teeth from braces or veneers, but strong, healthy teeth. Dr. Price photographed the faces and smiles of dozens of indigenous peoples. These were modern day Paleo tribes and they had beautiful teeth. The mouth and nose were large, allowing air to move freely. Tooth decay was absent and all teeth were accounted for.

You see, there was plenty of sugar and grain in the 1920's. Dr. Price saw horrible teeth and disease on a daily basis as a practicing dentist. He knew the cause was the current diet in the 1920's. He understood vitamin deficiencies play a major role in tooth decay. But he made a very interesting observation during his travels. When a Paleo person moved to live in the modern world (of the 1920's), their teeth began to rot just like the city people's did. Incredibly, when a Paleo women moved to a modern area with access to sugar and grain, she gave birth to a child who would develop a small mouth with crowded teeth and a small nose. Is this not the same as 21st century children's mouths? Crowded teeth waiting for an orthodontist to apply metal straightjackets? This is a perfect example of how poor nutrition can effect DNA. Similar genetics exist between mother and child, but the influence of nutrition and chemicals on the DNA is without a doubt.

★**LIVE WELL**: Poor nutrition leads to unhealthy teeth, which in turn can lead to an unhealthy heart.

ROOT OF THE CAUSE

If you were to create a scenario where bacteria were given permanent access to your blood stream, you couldn't do much better than a root canal. You see, every tooth is nourished by its root. This provides the blood supply to and from the tooth along with nerve fibers. Poor nutrition and chemicals can lead to a painful infection below the surface of the tooth. Could these same bacteria get access to your bloodstream and put your ticker at risk?

A dental procedure performed millions of times per year is the root canal. The root canal procedure destroys the nerve and blood supply, so you no longer feel pain. This is similar to someone hitting your toe with a hammer, but the doctor cuts off the nerve supply so you don't feel the pain. Dr. Hal Huggins realized microscopic roots still remain after the root canal and are a source of continuous infection. Infection and inflammation continue in a tooth that is essentially dead. That's right. You are living with a dead body part with ZERO ability to fight off infection because the blood supply is cut off. The immune system cannot get where it needs to go.

The *Journal of the American Dental Association* concluded in 2009, "Among participants with 25 or more teeth, those with a greater self-reported history of endodontic therapy were more likely to have coronary heart disease than were those reporting no history of endodontic therapy."[247] Endodontic therapy is treatment of the root, and the endodontists make a fortune performing root canals.

You must keep your teeth healthy. I have seen many patients with elevated markers of inflammation such as hs-CRP and myeloperoxidase, the source of which was a root canal tooth. In my experience, eliminating sugar, grain, and dairy from you diet can rid the body of inflammation and infections.

I know it is a big procedure, but the second option is to remove the root canal tooth. Usually it is only a cosmetic issue and the loss of the tooth does not affect chewing. I realize many patients house several root canal teeth. The choice is theirs, I am only writing this book to provide information. What someone does with the information is up to them. Once the area heals, the space can be left empty or a bridge or an implant may be used. In my opinion, I would think long and hard about an implant. This introduces another foreign and dead material into the body.

★**LIVE WELL**: It is important to keep your teeth healthy. Your mouth, and heart, will thank you.

METAL FILLINGS

Another issue near and dear to your friendly neighborhood dentist is metal amalgam. As mentioned in my chapter "Heavy Metal Madness," amalgams are toxic. Mercury is no longer in thermometers and a broken light bulb is a HAZMAT emergency, but it's okay to store mercury in your mouth? Amalgams are 50% mercury, some silver, plenty of tin, and other toxic metals. Many dentists refuse to believe amalgams are dangerous, but these docs are clearly in denial. True in cardiology and true in dentistry, it is a hard pill for a doctor to swallow, thinking they are causing patients harm.

If not metal amalgam, usually a plastic resin containing BPA is used. Remember our discussions about BPA throughout this book? It is a known cause of disease. There are other options with safer materials. Ask your holistic dentist. If you have a cavity and the doctor is recommending a filling, go Paleo immediately. You will notice a change overnight. If your teeth currently contain amalgams, find a holistic dentist to get them out. Your average dentist is not experienced with the safe removal of amalgams and will not be supportive of your decision. You need people on your health team who are in alignment with your beliefs. Detox and chelate immediately after the removal procedure. While the amalgams are in place, consume chlorella multiple times per day to bind metals.

★**LIVE WELL**: Find a holistic dentist to remove metal amalgams, and don't forget to detox and chelate!

KEEP YOUR MOUTH HEALTHY:
1. Eat Paleo and avoid chemicals. Do everything you can to keep your body healthy.
2. Brush daily, preferably after every meal. An electric toothbrush, although a source of EMF, may be the best way to clean your teeth.
3. Get rid of toxic toothpastes like Crest and Colgate. Use natural, fluoride-free toothpaste or use baking soda. Honestly, plain water on your brush is really all you need.

4. Floss your teeth daily to lower inflammation.[248]
5. Rinse your mouth with colloidal silver if you feel an infection brewing.

Seek out the opinion of a biologic dentist who practices safe dentistry. These doctors attempt to minimize the use of chemicals and suggest methods for detox before and after procedures. Some may even use herbal or homeopathic remedies for pain and infection control. Find a dentist who will not force you into routine dental x-rays, which are essentially worthless and subject you to serious radiation. Check out IAOMT.org or holisticdental.org for a doctor in your area.

★LIVE WELL: Throw out the chemicals and buy all-natural, fluoride-free toothpastes and mouthwashes.

CASE STUDY

Marcy was a 45 year old woman who felt like she was 85. Constantly in pain, she visited many doctors who labeled her with fibromyalgia, or as just plain crazy. After doing an in-depth history, my wife surmised Marcy's issue to be related to a chronic infection under a root canal tooth. Once blood tests demonstrated elevated markers of inflammation and very high LDL, the tooth had to go. Although it seemed drastic at the time, removal of the infected dead tooth was the answer to her health complaints and within three months, blood tests were normal.

ACTION PLAN

1. Avoid dental problems by getting rid of sugar from your diet.
2. Do not let children eat too much sugar.
3. Brush and floss daily.
4. Find a holistic dentist.
5. Remove the metal amalgams.
6. Skin the root canal. If the tooth cannot be saved, you need to have it extracted.

Chapter 16

TOP TWENTY SUPPLEMENTS

"The best time to plant a tree was 20 years ago, the second best time is now."
—Chinese Proverb

A sk 100 doctors if vitamins work. You will get a variety of answers and opinions. Most will scoff at the idea, some will shrug their shoulders like there may be some benefit, and a few will be enthusiastic. The truth is medical doctors receive ZERO training in vitamins, minerals, botanicals, and other natural remedies. We are trained to shun anything but pills and procedures. I worked in the hospital for over 16 years. The number of vitamin overdoses I saw? Zero.

Do not go at it alone. Find a holistic doctor to guide you, as supplements are very complicated. Genetic tests are valuable to help determine the type of vitamin and quantity to take. There are some excellent companies performing high-end tests with valuable information. Your natural doctor is experienced in interpreting these tests. Invest in your health.

I am not a "crazy cardiologist." I am a board certified cardiologist recommending proven natural supplements instead of prescribing poison to achieve health. You decide who the real "quacks" are.

The following is my top 20 supplements for heart health. All of these products and more can be purchased on our website, TheDrsWolfson.com. We sourced the best quality supplements so follow the doctors you can trust.

Please understand there will never be a head to head comparison of Lipitor versus berberine, or fish oil versus aspirin. Since vitamins and natural supplements cannot be patented, no one is going to invest money to study them. This leaves the door open for the skeptic to criticize natural remedies. Fortunately, there are thousands of papers proving vitamins do work! Take a look.

1. MULTIVITAMINS

I am often asked if a multivitamin is necessary. My answer is a resounding "Yes." A quality multivitamin will contain the foundation for a healthy supplement regimen and a healthy life. Too often, patients are taking high doses of a few vitamins, yet are horribly depleted in others. For example, many people take zinc to boost their immune system. Zinc consumption leads to copper loss. Calcium tablets are taken like candy, but can be dangerous without proper vitamin K consumption. A multivitamin helps to make sure all the bases are covered.

From the *Journal of the American College of Nutrition* in 2013 comes a review of multivitamin studies. The conclusion is that multivitamins decrease overall mortality and appear to lower cardiovascular and cancer risk.[249] Another recent study revealed improved brain function in those assigned a multivitamin.[250] The *Journal of the American Medical Association (JAMA)* also published a study showing multivitamins significantly reduced the incidence of cancers in men.[251]

There are some studies that did not find a benefit of multivitamins, but these trials usually use cheap vitamins in low doses and get published in journals funded by Big Pharma. To me, it just makes sense a multivitamin ensures you are getting each nutrient. Many believe diet alone provides enough vitamin and mineral support. This myth is perpetuated when certain foods are labeled as a "complete source" of nutrients. But the government's recommended daily allowance (RDA) is the MINIMUM required to prevent disease. This is not good enough. We want to thrive, not just survive. For example, the RDA of vitamin C is 90mg. This tiny amount is nothing compared to studies showing doses 20-50 times higher are needed. Linus Pauling used doses 500 times higher to prove benefits for certain conditions. Pauling won the Nobel Prize, twice!

Chapters of this book were devoted to the problems with the Standard American Diet (SAD). Most people exist on fast food; toxins in a bag that at best provide the minimum nutrition to prevent overt illness. These "foods" are void of many vitamins and minerals. In fact, most food labels include data on nutrition content before the food was processed and cooked. Cheap vitamins are added to grains and dairy, but these are clearly inferior forms. The consumption of certain foods and drink actually causes us to lose vitamins and minerals, including calcium, magnesium, and zinc. Pharmaceuticals are notorious for causing nutrient depletion, including B vitamins, minerals, and CoQ10. Metformin, a common diabetes drug, causes B12 depletion. All statin drugs deplete CoQ10.

Even those of us who eat the best organic diets are held captive by nutrient-depleted soil. Reliance on fertilizer, which only replaces nitrogen, potassium, and phosphorus, is leading consumers to micronutrient deficiency. Plants will grow, but the nutritional value is gone. Man will never be able to duplicate Mother Nature's perfect soil. Food from 10,000 years ago grew naturally in the area and climate from which it was native. Broccoli, kale, and other greens grew only in select regions where the soil in the area was perfect for that food.

Thousands of years ago, the air, land, and water were pure, leading to amazing vegetation. Today, pollution has ruined the skies and the streams. Pollutants kill the good bacteria in the ground. The negative effects of this are limitless. There are valid concerns that the shipping of produce over long distances allows for nutrient decay. Picking unripe fruit results in diminished vitamin content. Antioxidants, such as polyphenols and carotenoids, are not produced until the fruit is naturally ripened on the tree, bush, or vine. Food storage and cooking can lead to vitamin loss. The best way to store food is in glass, yet light can destroy vitamins and phytonutrients.

We formulated an incredible MULTI from the finest ingredients, without harmful fillers. Activated B vitamins are in our product. Plenty of magnesium and potassium are in our MULTI, along with lithium, a nutrient missing from soil, but beneficial for brain health. Our MULTI is the perfect foundation for a healthy supplement regimen.

2. GREENS POWDER

I start off every day with a greens drink. Nothing is healthier than fresh green juice made in your own home or local juice bar. Just make sure the juice is made from 100% organic produce. It boggles my mind how people choose to drink juice made from pesticide produce. Concentrating pesticides from non-organic produce into a juice has devastating health consequences. Another option is a powder made from dehydrated organic vegetables. Just add water and breakfast is served. I prefer this to capsules because a drink is more like a meal. The cost of this supplement should be considered as part of your food budget. Heather and I developed an organic greens powder packaged in a glass bottle. Greens powder may be added to a protein shake and even added to salad. This is less expensive than a fresh juice, and you can travel with it easily.

The health benefits are obvious. You are getting multiple servings of vegetables with a multitude of vitamins and minerals. The greens drink is a blast of antioxidants, which boost immunity and protect the heart and brain. These products alone reduced inflammation in many of my patients.

But don't just take my word for it. A 2013 study found powdered greens decrease inflammation and oxidation versus placebo. The levels of oxidized LDL, a major cause of blockages, were decreased.[252] Another trial found total cholesterol and circulation were improved in those participants who drank a greens powder supplement versus a placebo.[253] Greens powders work!

3. CHLORELLA AND SPIRULINA

Chlorella is nature's detoxifier. This fresh-water algae has been on the planet for two billion years, and is a natural way to clean the body and the blood of toxic heavy metals. Chlorella provides tremendous amounts of nourishment in addition to detoxifying the body and blood. This little green guy is loaded with protein, more than beef on a per-gram basis. Chlorella contains a hefty dose of vitamin A and significant amounts of vitamins B, C and E. It's packed with biotin, PABA and inositol. It has lots of iron and zinc and other minerals. You'll also find omega-3 fatty acids in chlorella (but not EPA and DHA, see below). A number of clinical studies on humans and animals found chlorella:

- Cuts the risk of cardiovascular disease.
- Improves cholesterol, triglycerides, and blood sugar.[254]
- Improves blood pressure control.
- Boosts your immune system.
- Slows cognitive decline.[255]
- Detoxifies heavy metals.
- Detoxifies insecticides and other chemicals.
- Reduces radiation damage.

Chlorella is one of nature's best sources for moving toxins from your body, toxins like mercury, arsenic and lead. Left unchecked, these heavy metals wreak havoc on your immune system. Metals will destroy the body unless steps are taken to assist with their removal. Chlorophyll binds to heavy metals and removes them from the body by excretion in stool. This process is called chelation. Chlorella is the perfect way to cleanse your liver and bowels and clear your blood of toxins. Chlorella contains high levels of chlorophyll, which is the molecule responsible for turning sunlight into usable plant energy.[256]

Spirulina is a tiny algae consumed as a food in powder or freeze-dried form. This powerhouse has been proven to prevent disease and to maintain good health. It contains a load of protein along with nutrients like iron, vitamins A, K, and B complex, as well as a generous supply of carotenoids with antioxidant properties such as beta-carotene and yellow xanthophyll. Spirulina also has fatty acids and nucleic acids to maintain cellular health and integrity.

Some of the health benefits of Spirulina include:

- **Boosts the immune system**—an animal study from Taiwan demonstrated spirulina supports a healthy immune system. Spirulina contains nutrients like zinc, copper, iron, manganese, selenium, and chromium. One study showed spirulina helps with allergies by reducing nasal discharge, congestion, sneezing and itching.

- **Slashes cancer risks**—a study in China showed selenium-infused spirulina inhibited the growth of MCF-7 breast cancer cells.
- **Normalizes cholesterol levels**—Elderly patients given spirulina improved cholesterol levels over those given a placebo.
- **Reduces risks of stroke**—An animal study in India found spirulina had a protective effect on the nervous system and brain of rats exposed to high amounts of free radicals, which indicates spirulina may be effective in stroke prevention.

Ten mixed carotenoids make spirulina the richest beta-carotene food. These carotenoids work together to increase antioxidant protection. Its beta-carotene is ten times more concentrated than carrots. This helps with healthy eyes and vision, and many consider it the ideal anti-aging food. Spirulina was awarded a patent in Russia in 1994 as a medical food to reduce allergic reactions from radiation sickness. Its unique combination of phytonutrients, such as chlorophyll, help cleanse our bodies of toxic chemicals.[257]

Heather and I formulated our Cardio Superfood to contain 50% organic chlorella and 50% spirulina. We recommend it after seafood, after a workout, after the sauna, and any time you want a quick detox.

4. OMEGA-3

Omega-3 oil is part of a healthy diet and supplement regimen. It is another supplement in our arsenal to combat disease, with hundreds of trials documenting benefit for asthma, allergies, eczema, dementia, depression, and arthritis, to name only a few. This polyunsaturated fat is critically important for brain, heart, and total body health.

In 1999, the GISSI-Prevention trial was published, and included 11,000 patients with a recent heart attack. They were put on one gram of omega-3 fish oil or placebo and were followed for 3.5 years. Amazingly, the omega-3 group had a 20% lower risk of death. Other studies demonstrate the more omega-3 in your cells, the less likely a heart attack or stroke. Multiple studies find omega-3 improves blood pressure control.[258]

The quality of the omega is of critical importance. Many people try using a nut or seed source of omega-3 such as flax or walnut oil. Unfortunately, the body does not convert this form into DHA and EPA, the necessary omega-3 type for health. You must choose a product that contains EPA and DHA. Some of the best heart data comes from the high DHA variety. It doesn't really matter if you use fish oil, krill oil, or algae oil. What matters is boosting your omega-3 index. Take a multivitamin along with the omega-3 oil for anti-oxidants and assimilation. Omega-3 oils are best stored in the refrigerator to prevent oxidation damage. Cellular levels of omega should be assessed to assure integration into the cell membrane. This is a simple blood test.

5. COQ10

If you are looking to find a source for energy along with cardiovascular benefits, look no further than CoQ10. I know it is a strange name for a critical nutrient, but don't dismiss it. At a basic level, CoQ10 is made up of hydrogen, carbon, and oxygen. Nothing fancy, just those three atoms. You see, the energy furnace of the cell is called the mitochondria. Most cells contain hundreds of these fuel factories. Without mitochondria, the energy currency of the body, ATP, cannot be formed. CoQ10 is plentiful in the mitochondria.

CoQ10 is found in the human body in two forms, ubiquinone and ubiquinol. Debate rages on about which form is better. The simple answer is both have utility, with ubiquinone better for people younger than forty and ubiquinol for those older than forty. Ubiquinol is an excellent antioxidant and free radical scavenger. It often travels around the body inside the LDL particle and protects the particle from damage. Ubiquinone is cheaper and may be a better option for those on a budget.

In a study presented to the European Society of Cardiology in 2013, CoQ10 supplements improved survival in patients with heart failure. Furthermore, the nutrient decreased hospitalizations and improved symptoms as compared to those patients using only a placebo. After two years, cardiovascular events occurred in 14% of patients in the CoQ10 group versus 25 % of patients in the placebo group. With regard to all-cause mortality at two years, 9% of patients had died in the CoQ10 group compared to 17% in the placebo group. That is very impressive data. The latest meta-analysis out of Tulane University, which pooled results from thirteen studies involving 395 heart failure patients, found CoQ10 increased ejection fraction (a measurement of heart function) by an average of 3.67%.[259]

CoQ10 is fat-soluble and is best absorbed with a meal. Dosing can range from 50mg on up to over 1000mg in divided doses depending on the medical condition. As we get older, the production of CoQ10 decreases. Several pharmaceuticals, such as statins and beta-blockers, also decrease levels. In fact, statins may reduce CoQ10 levels by 40% and supplementation may prevent statin-induced muscle damage.[260] Those who perform strenuous exercise also benefit from CoQ10 supplementation.

6. VITAMIN K

Most people understand vitamin D is critical to health but know little of vitamin K, the little orphan Annie of the fat-soluble group. Vitamin D promotes the uptake of calcium and keeps it floating around the blood, but it is vitamin K that stores calcium in bone and teeth. Without K, calcium deposits everywhere in the body, including blood vessels and coronary plaque. Warfarin (Coumadin), a pharmaceutical that inhibits vitamin K activity, is linked to osteoporosis risk and to accelerated coronary calcification.[261]

Vitamin K is a fat-soluble vitamin, along with A, D, and E. As such, it travels around the body bound inside the LDL molecule and other lipoproteins (notice the importance of LDL). Vitamin K is involved with many enzyme functions and is famous for its role in the blood-clotting cascade. Without K you will bleed, but additional K does not increase clotting risk.

Vitamin K is found as K1 and K2. K1 is synthesized by plants and found in high concentration in green leafy vegetables. K2 is the main storage form in the body and can be formed from conversion of K1, produced by bacteria in the large intestine (another reason to take probiotics), or ingested from other animal sources. K1 is critical to blood clotting; K2 for cardiovascular protection, cancer, and strong bones.

Benefits of vitamin K2:

- Reduced risk of coronary artery disease.[262]
- Lowers blood pressure.[263]
- Lowers inflammation.[264]
- Improves blood sugar control.[265]
- Lowers cancer risk.[266]
- Decreases mortality.[267]
- Keeps calcium in bones and out of arteries.

The best way to get vitamins K1 and K2 is through food. Eat Paleo and you will be covered. For those who take vitamin D supplements, a K2 supplement is imperative. The more D you take, the more K you need. My rule of thumb is 50 mcg of K2 as MK-7 for every 5000 of vitamin D3. For those with coronary disease or a strong family history, at least 100mcg should be consumed daily. Speak with your doctor about vitamin K if you take warfarin.

7. VITAMIN E

Vitamin E has been touted as a supplement critical to health. It is necessary for skeletal, cardiac, and smooth muscle maintenance. Two groups, tocopherols and tocotrienols, and eight types make up this important substance. Of the eight vitamin E types, gamma tocopherol is most commonly found in food. Nuts, seeds, olives, green veggies, and avocado are high in vitamin E content. Many oils are also loaded with vitamin E with my favorites coming from almonds and walnuts.

As a powerful antioxidant, vitamin E safeguards your body from free-radical damage and various chronic illnesses including cardiovascular disease. Many population studies find those subjects with higher vitamin E levels are at lower risk of developing heart disease. A large study suggested postmenopausal women who eat vitamin-E-rich diets might reduce their risk of fatal strokes.[268]

Get these benefits from Vitamin E:

- Improves vascular endothelial function.[269]
- Protects cell membranes from free-radical damage.[270]
- Contains anticlotting properties.[271]

- Defends against oxidative damage, which can cause heart disease.[272]
- Reduces CRP, an inflammatory protein linked to heart disease.[273]
- May prevent atrial fibrillation.[274]
- Vitamin E supplements may reduce Alzheimer's disease progression.[275]
- Finally, low levels of vitamin E can lead to increased bone fracture risk.[276]

Despite many positive conclusions, some studies do not find health benefits from vitamin E supplementation. One study found vitamin E increases prostate cancer risk, while another demonstrates protection from prostate cancer. These mixed results are likely from using inferior, single-source supplements instead of high-quality mixed versions.

To gain vitamin E's full benefits, you need to ingest all eight of its health-enhancing compounds (alpha, beta, gamma and delta in tocopherol and tocotrienol groups). Compare labels carefully when you shop for a vitamin E supplement. Choose one that combines all or most types. A formula containing only alpha tocopherol may deplete your body's supply of other healthy tocopherols and tocotrienols. Try to find a brand of vitamin E without a capsule full of soybean oil. Rice bran oil would be my preference.

Oral vitamin E dosages range from 20 to 1000 IU (international units). For disease prevention and treatment, adult clinical trial participants typically took 400 to 800 IU per day.

8. VITAMIN C

The list of benefits of vitamin C is very long. From heart health to immune boosting, this nutrient is a winner. Many trials reveal blood pressure is reduced with vitamin C supplementation. In fact, one study found blood pressure was 20 points lower in the vitamin C group versus the placebo group.[277] This nutrient makes pharmaceuticals more effective at reducing blood pressure. A diuretic effect is also noted, therefore reducing leg swelling. A recent review of 44 trials found vitamin C, at doses above 500mg per day, improves endothelial function. If the cells lining the arteries are working, it is a good thing. Vitamin C lowers cholesterol, decreases LDL oxidation damage, decreases clotting, and lowers cardiovascular risk.[278] Vitamin C also improves sympathovagal tone, an effect that could reduce heart rhythm problems and improve symptoms in those people with light-headedness. Vitamin C lowers the risk of atrial fibrillation.[279] Blood vessels are made from collagen, a protein fiber dependent on vitamin C. I personally take two grams of C daily and increase up to 10 grams daily as needed for an immune boost.[280] Monthly intravenous vitamin C is also beneficial.

9. VITAMIN D

Low levels of vitamin D are associated with just about every disease, including coronary, stroke, hypertension, Alzheimer's, osteoporosis, and cancer. Getting sunshine is the best source of vitamin D, but it is often not possible in colder climates during the wintertime. One study found vitamin D plus calcium dropped systolic blood pressure by almost 10%.[281] I typically do not recommend calcium supplementation as you will read in a few pages.

Most studies use a cheap form of the vitamin as a stand-alone nutrient. We should not be taking any vitamins without a multivitamin as the base to the supplement regimen. It stands to reason vitamin D alone is not responsible for any actions, as a plethora of nutrients are necessary to accomplish health. The natural community has always strived for a blood level of 50. Monitoring serum calcium is useful to gauge if the vitamin D level is too high. If you take vitamin D, you should always take vitamin K2.

10. DIGESTIVE ENZYMES

You can't obtain the nutrients from food if you do not absorb them. You can't absorb the nutrients if you can't break down the food. Enter digestive enzymes: As we get older, our amount of stomach acid actually decreases, as do our digestive enzymes. The gut is the source of the majority of inflammation. If food is not digested appropriately, large food particles remain and irritate the lining of the intestines. This leads to a leaky gut, a situation where food and bacteria are able to get into the body where they do not belong. Now the immune system is activated and inflammation becomes rampant. All of this serves to increase cardiovascular risk.

Most people need to supplement betaine HCL and/or ox bile in addition to the digestive enzymes amylase, protease, and lipase. Reflux, or GERD, is a made-up disease that is easy to fix with nutrition and supplements. Hundreds of times, I have stopped the dangerous pharmaceuticals that inhibit acid production, and started my patients on natural therapies. My patients enjoy tremendous results and are able to heal their bodies. Speak with your natural doctor to find out how you can improve your digestive health.

11. BERBERINE

Berberine may turn out to be one of the best supplements of all! This botanical extract has received a lot of attention over the last few years for its incredible health benefits. Studies demonstrate an improvement in lipid control, diabetes prevention, heart failure, weight loss, and memory. Millions of people have the Metabolic Syndrome, which includes lipid abnormalities, hypertension, fatty liver, and elevated blood sugar. Berberine is proven to help control this condition.[282]

AMPK and Berberine

An enzyme is a protein that turns product A into product B. There is a very important enzyme called AMPK, which is the master switch when it comes to cellular energy. When this AMPK is activated, good things happen such as improved cholesterol, glucose, and energy. Berberine (and resveratrol) activates the AMPK enzyme.[283] Berberine lowers inflammation and improves vascular endothelial function. It basically leads to blood vessel expansion, therefore increasing blood flow. The diabetes medicine metformin activates AMPK, and berberine is just as effective when it comes to blood sugar control, without the side effects.[284] A recent meta-analysis combined data from 14 randomized trials involving 1,068 participants. Treatment with both berberine and lifestyle modification showed significant blood sugar and lipid benefits. Effects were similar to those obtained by the standard diabetes drugs metformin, glipizide, and rosiglitazone.[285] Wouldn't you rather take a supplement from a rain-forest versus something made in a laboratory test-tube?

Lipid Profile

In 2004, an article described how berberine reduced triglycerides by 35% and LDL-cholesterol by 25%.[286] Oxidation damage occurs to LDL causing it to become a toxic molecule, which easily enters the blood vessel wall. This can be prevented by berberine.[287] In a 2011 trial of sixty patients with fatty liver disease, berberine demonstrated a 70% improvement in liver ultrasounds. Triglycerides decreased significantly in this trial.[288] A 2010 trial was done with berberine in sixty patients with type-2 diabetes. The berberine group had significantly lower levels of free fatty acids, chemicals that are toxic to the pancreas and linked with insulin resistance. Free fatty acids are easily measured on standard blood tests.[289] Berberine can be combined with plant sterols for a synergistic effect.[290]Although I am not a proponent of statins, berberine combined with statins improved the lipid profile more than either product alone.[291] Berberine improves arterial endothelial function and suppresses pro-inflammatory cytokines.[292]

A July 2003 study published in the *American Journal of Cardiology* examined the use of berberine in congestive heart failure (CHF). The authors divided 156 CHF patients into two groups. All patients were treated with typical drug therapy, but one group was also given berberine at a dose of 1.2 to 2.0 grams per day. After eight weeks of berberine treatment, there was a significantly greater increase in ejection fraction, exercise capacity, improvement of the dyspnea-fatigue index, and a decrease in PVCs [premature ventricular complexes] compared with the control group. Mortality was decreased in the berberine-treated patients during long-term follow-up (7 patients receiving treatment died vs. 13 on placebo). Pro-arrhythmia was not observed, and there were no apparent side effects.[293]

Berberine is a winner. Dosing is 500mg 2-3x per day with or without food. I created an amazing supplement combining berberine with other beneficial nutrients.

12. HAWTHORN

Hawthorn is a thorny tree found in various regions around the world. People realized its heart benefits many years ago. Hawthorn:

- Improves LDL numbers
- Lowers triglycerides
- Enhances cholesterol degradation to bile acids
- Promotes bile flow
- Suppresses cholesterol biosynthesis
- Inhibits the angiotensin converting enzyme (ACE)
- Serves as a mild diuretic
- Coronary vasodilator—suppresses the production of endothelin-1
- Improves edema
- Improves ejection fraction (EF)
- Improves symptoms and exercise performance
- Decreased mortality by 20% in patients with EF 25-35%[294]

13. L-ARGININE/ L-CITRULLINE

L-citrulline is an amino acid originally isolated from watermelon rinds. Years of studying this protein building block led to some interesting findings. In a recent study, men with mild erectile dysfunction received a placebo for 1 month and L-citrulline, 1.5 g/d, for another month. A total of 24 patients, mean age 57, finished the study without adverse events. An improvement in the erection hardness score occurred in 50% of the men taking L-citrulline and only 8% of the men when taking placebo. The average number of intercourses per month doubled in the treatment group.[295] While L-citrulline may not be as powerful as the little blue pill, it is safe, cheap, and effective.

There are cardiovascular benefits of L-citrulline. A study was done on 35 heart failure patients randomized into two groups: an experimental group, with oral L-citrulline supplementation (3 g/day) and a control group. In the experimental group, the left ventricular ejection fraction (measure of heart function) increased by 20%. In addition, heart failure symptoms markedly improved in 35%.[296] Another study found a combination of the amino acids citrulline and arginine improves endothelial function and blood pressure in patients with congestive heart failure.[297]

L-arginine is another amino acid used by many people looking for natural remedies to hypertension, erectile dysfunction, and angina. It is a vasodilator that opens up blood vessels, but the problem is that when taken orally, L-arginine is broken down by the body before it can really start working. In contrast, L-citrulline escapes this breakdown and is then converted to L-arginine. L-citrulline is excellent for muscle recovery after exercise and may even enhance athletic performance.[298]

14. MAGNESIUM

Magnesium is an element abundantly found in soil and is the fourth most common element on earth behind iron, oxygen, and silicon. Seawater also contains a lot of magnesium. Magnesium is so critical to health; it is found at the center of chlorophyll, the protein in plants that harnesses the energy of the sun. Magnesium is involved in over 300 enzymatic reactions in the body.

Some functions of magnesium include:

- Production and utilization of fat, protein, and carbohydrates, along with DNA.
- Cell division and growth.
- Immune support and inflammation regulation.
- Maintenance of sodium and fluid balance.
- Muscle contraction and relaxation.
- Cellular communication.

Most people are deficient in magnesium for a variety of reasons:

1. The typical SAD diet (Standard American Diet) of fast food and sugar snacks washed down by soda does not contain much in the way of nutrition, let alone sufficient magnesium. White flour, white rice, and white sugar are void in magnesium. Additionally, magnesium is used up in many of the reactions to digest carbohydrates and sugar, therefore is not available for other basic body functions.
2. The amount of magnesium in the soil where even the best organic vegetables grow is limited. After years of farming, so many of the vital minerals are gone. In fact, a study from the *Journal of the American College*

of Nutrition revealed a 40% drop in the nutrient content of vegetables since 1950![299] Another reason to consume a quality multivitamin.

3. Caffeinated beverages like coffee, tea, and soda produce a diuretic effect causing mineral loss through urine. Alcohol also wastes magnesium. Our ancestors drank spring water, well water, or water from streams and rivers, thus enjoying the high mineral content of those sources. Lastly, the phosphoric acid in soda binds magnesium in the gut, and is therefore not absorbed.

4. Pharmaceuticals cause nutrient loss, led by diuretics that waste magnesium, calcium, and potassium. I check intracellular levels of these minerals in my patients, and they are low the vast majority of the time.

5. Society is crazed with the idea that supplemental calcium prevents osteoporosis and fractures (not true). Therefore, everyone and their mother load up on calcium, which leads to a magnesium deficiency. Paleo people consumed magnesium to calcium at a 2:1 ratio.

6. Chronic stress leads to magnesium depletion. The constant release of neurotransmitters, such as norepinephrine and dopamine along with the hormone cortisol, depletes magnesium. The deficiency of magnesium leads to anxiety, sleep loss, and depression.

Magnesium supplements:
- Lower blood pressure.[300]
- Raise HDL.[301]
- Lower triglycerides.[302]
- Lower CRP (a measure of inflammation).[303]
- Improve blood sugar control.[304]

There are many different types of magnesium such as citrate, malate, and glycinate. Each form is associated with different health claims according to medical authorities. All are beneficial except magnesium oxide. This version is cheap and poorly absorbed. Magnesium gel, cream, and oil are other ways to absorb this nutrient.

Check with your doctor to see if magnesium supplementation is right for you. Patients with kidney disease need close monitoring. The main side effect of oral magnesium is diarrhea, so you may need to back off a little.

15. PROBIOTICS

Probiotic literally means "pro-life," and antibiotic means "anti-life." Doctors use the term probiotic to encompass the trillions of bacteria that colonize our intestines. The GI tract has a delicate balance of beneficial and harmful bacteria doing the dance every day. When this coexistence gets out of whack in favor of the bad guys, symptoms and disease will start. The organs from the mouth to the rectum are of utmost importance to our health. Damage anywhere along that route will lead to disease.

When our ancestors wanted a carrot, they would pull one out of the ground and eat it. In present day, our store bought vegetables are pre-washed before we buy them, then usually scrubbed at home to get off any dirt remnants. I am not opposed to washing off our food due to toxic soil, air, water, and the hands of those who handled the food. This is all the more reason to consume probiotics on a daily basis. In addition, our hands used to be dirty from the soil during our hunter-gatherer lives. Not any longer. You can't walk five feet without running into hand sanitizer, which effectively removes all good probiotics along with giving you an extra dose of chemicals that lead to cancer and disrupt hormones. Could many diseases afflicting our children, and the recurrent infections we all seem to get, be due to our sterilized society?

Poor nutrition from grain (especially gluten containing grains), dairy, and sugar wreak havoc on the gut and can allow the bad bacteria and fungi to flourish. Antibiotics and steroids are major offenders, as are allergenic foods. Also, genetically modified foods will surely alter our intestinal flora, as will fluoride and chlorine. Lastly, if your digestion is limited from inadequate amounts of stomach acid and digestive enzymes, disease will begin.

The health benefits of probiotics have been known for thousands of years. Our ancestors had no idea about the tiny bacteria themselves, but they knew the healing properties of fermented foods such as sauerkraut, kimchi, kefir, and yogurt. One bite of these foods has trillions of good bacteria and I recommend eating kraut and/or kimchi weekly. I am talking about raw, living sauerkraut from a company like Rejuvenative Foods, not the garbage variety at a typical delicatessen. Kombucha tea is another excellent source of probiotics.

Why does a cardiologist care about probiotics? Cardiovascular disease is a result of toxins leading to inflammation, and a major source of inflammation is the gut. Heal the gut and heal the heart. A study in the *European Journal of Clinical Nutrition* found those patients randomly assigned to probiotics increased their HDL from 50 to 62. Probiotics may also reduce blood pressure. A 2015 study found heart failure patient's ejection fraction improved from 39% to 46% with the use of probiotics.[305] This improvement is on par with any pharmaceutical.

In addition, probiotics:

- Aid in food digestion and may reduce reflux symptoms.
- Enhance the synthesis of B vitamins and improve calcium absorption.
- Improve symptoms of irritable bowel syndrome and ulcerative colitis.
- (In women) Promote vaginal and urinary health.
- Support immune function.
- May inhibit antibiotic-associated, and Traveler's, diarrhea.
- Improve your breath.

It's good to take a variety of probiotics, as there are hundreds of different strains that inhabit a healthy gastrointestinal tract. You cannot overdose on probiotics. Side effects are mostly limited to loose stools. Read the label for information about taking with food or on an empty stomach. The Drs. Wolfson brand can be consumed either way.

16. TAURINE

Want to be strong like a bull? Take taurine, the nutrient with many different functions. Taurine is found in animal tissues, and is a major constituent of bile, the digestive juice critical for breaking down food in your gut. In fact, taurine comes from the Latin word taurus, which means bull or ox, as it was first isolated from ox bile in 1827. Most of the production of taurine occurs in the pancreas from the amino acid cysteine. This is one of many reasons to maintain a healthy pancreas; therefore, avoid sugar and alcohol— two items that damage this organ.

A study from 1988 in the *American Journal of Clinical Nutrition* revealed vegans are woefully low in taurine, another knock against this unnatural diet. Animal products like meat and seafood are known to be excellent sources of taurine. Breast milk is high in taurine, highlighting its importance. If babies need it, we likely need it. Boosting your intake of the amino acid cysteine, the precursor to taurine, is beneficial and is found in liver, eggs, and other meat cuts. Garlic, onions, broccoli, and Brussel sprouts also contain plenty of cysteine.

Some of the benefits of taurine include:

- Lowers blood pressure in hypertensive people.[306]
- Improves cholesterol by increasing bile secretion.[307]
- Increases hepatic LDL receptors.[308]
- Improves heart function.[309]
- Improves heart failure symptoms.[310]
- Improves exercise capacity.[311]
- Improves endothelial function (in rats).[312]
- Acts as an antioxidant.[313]

Taurine also reduces extra heartbeats known as PVC's by 50%. Many people experience these symptoms as palpitations or thumps in their chest. By combining taurine with L-arginine, the PVC's totally stopped.[314] Taurine may also prevent damage from diabetes and elevated blood sugar. Lastly, taurine easily crosses the blood-brain barrier and can improve mood and lower anxiety. Many natural supplements used for anxiety and depression contain this nutrient. Taking taurine supplements is easy and surprisingly affordable. I recommend my patients to start off on 1000mg of taurine 2x per day. Some people need higher doses, up to 6000mg per day. I am not aware of any data regarding overdose levels of taurine, but most studies conclude the 6000mg as a therapeutic amount. It comes in capsules or powder. The powder can be added to smoothies, juice, water, or greens drinks.

I am very successful in my practice at getting people off pharmaceuticals for high blood pressure and cholesterol. Inflammation markers are easily improved. My patients with heart failure are usually able to safely stop the drugs. Taurine is always part of a healthy supplements regimen to achieve these goals.

17. GARLIC

This plant is known as the "stinking rose" for a reason. But if you can handle the odor, this becomes one heck of a beneficial supplement. I find the healthier one eats, the less of an odor garlic creates. Many cultures throughout history recognized garlic's health value and used it in cooking. Today, garlic gives great flavor to many dishes, but it can also be found in supplement form, providing medicinal value.[315]

Cardiovascular (and other) benefits:

- Reduces plaque formation
- Lowers blood pressure
- Decreases LDL particles
- Decreases LDL oxidation
- Lowers triglycerides
- Inhibits platelet aggregation
- Increases fibrinolytic activity
- Lowers blood sugar
- Anti-cancer
- Anti-microbial
- Chelates

18. BEETROOT POWDER

Those red things often used as a garnish pack incredible health benefits. Beetroot is a dark red vegetable that grows underground. The leaves are above the surface and contain plenty of nutrients. But be careful, the leaves consumed in excess can lead to some serious detoxification effects, similar to the flu. Trust me, I know first-hand.

According to the USDA, beetroot is an excellent source of fiber, folate, magnesium, potassium, iron, and zinc. The beet greens are very high in vitamin K. There are many ways to consume beets, but the best way is raw. They can be shredded into salad, cut in slices like chips and dipped into guacamole, or juiced. Fermented beets are another tasty treat. Cooking may change some of the nutrient composition. Steaming is the best way to cook. If you boil beets, drink the leftover water.

Health Benefits of Beetroot:

1. Reduce blood pressure because they contain nitrates, which are vasodilators.[316]
2. Reduce homocysteine since beetroots are high in betaine, and convert homocysteine to methionine.[317] Elevated homocysteine is a risk factor for just about disease.
3. Improve endothelial function, which leads to healthier blood vessels.[318]
4. Improve athletic performance.[319]
5. Improve blood sugar control.[320]
6. Improve peripheral artery circulation.[321]
7. Provide tremendous antioxidant supply that limits free radical damage in the body.[322]
8. Inhibit platelet function, and act as a natural blood thinner.[323]

Some of the studies that discovered these incredible benefits were done using beetroot powder. Beetroot powder should be organic or at least GMO free. Beetroot powder goes really well with a morning smoothie or greens drink. Start off at ½ teaspoon, 2x per day and increase as tolerated.

Beets will turn your urine and stool red, so be ready. Many people panic and think they are bleeding internally, when beets are the actual culprit. Once again, beets are very detoxifying, so be cautious and start slow. If you are on a sugar-free cleanse, you may want to skip the beets, which are a little high in sugar.

19. NATTOKINASE

Looking for the key ingredient to the longevity of the Japanese? It may be nattokinase.

Nattokinase (pronounced nat-oh-KY-nase) is an enzyme extracted from a Japanese food called Natto. For thousands of years, the Japanese enjoyed this food from fermented soybeans. Nattokinase is produced by a bacterium acting on the soybeans.

So what makes this enzyme so beneficial? It works as a natural clot buster and blood thinner. My patients who take nattokinase all admit to easy bruising and prolonged bleeding if they cut themselves. Out of hundreds of people on nattokinase, I have never seen a serious bleeding event, quite the contrast to aspirin and other prescription blood thinners. No large trials compare nattokinase to drugs like aspirin and warfarin (Coumadin), but I will share some data.

Nattokinase:

1. Decreases blood clotting.[324]
2. Inhibits platelet aggregation.[325]
3. Decreases amyloid plaque in dementia.[326]

I recommend nattokinase to my patients with:

1. A history of coronary artery disease for use instead of aspirin
2. Atrial fibrillation
3. A history of deep vein thrombosis (DVT) or pulmonary embolism (PE)
4. Elevated Lp(a)
5. Several risk factors for coronary artery disease

The dose of nattokinase is 100mg, 2 times per day away from food, as food can inhibit its absorption. Some people may need 3 times per day dosing. An alternative to nattokinase is lumbrokinase. Some prefer it to nattokinase as a way to avoid soy.

As always, check with your doctor to see if natural blood thinners are for you.

20. RED YEAST RICE (RYR)

Cholesterol is a critical molecule in the body and its importance was discussed extensively in this book. But there may be a point where LDL levels are too high, especially in patients with a history of coronary artery disease such as a heart attack, stent, or bypass procedure. If you are following Paleo and taking appropriate supplements, but LDL particles are above 2000 AND you have a history of coronary disease, RYR may be a good option. It is usually well tolerated.

RYR is a product of rice fermented with a yeast called Monascus purpureus, giving the supplement a bright reddish purple color. The original statin drug formula came from red yeast rice. RYR may cause similar side effects as statins, so this supplement should be monitored closely.

Here are some of the proven benefits:[327]

1. Lowers LDL (up to 30%)
2. Lowers hs-CRP (a marker of inflammation)
3. Decreases leptin
4. Raises adiponectin
5. Appears to be safe in people with statin intolerance
6. Lowers Lp(a)
7. Lowers heart attack risk in those with a previous heart attack

Look for a citrinin-free product. Citrinin is a toxin found in yeast that can lead to kidney damage. Dosing ranges from 1200mg to 4800mg at bedtime. I recommend 100mg of CoQ10 at least 2 times per day if you take red yeast rice, given its statin similarity.

WHAT ABOUT CALCIUM?

For years, millions of women swallowed calcium supplements with the goal of preventing osteoporosis. Even the makers of Tums advertise it as a great source of calcium for osteoporosis prevention. The benefit is very small, if any. The problem with most studies is that calcium was used in isolation without vitamins D, K, and other bone-building nutrients. Most trials using calcium plus D failed to show a lower fracture rate.

Might calcium supplements increase cardiovascular disease risk? That was the subject of the European Prospective Investigation into Cancer and Nutrition study (EPIC-Heidelberg). This study found those patients taking calcium supplements had DOUBLE the risk of heart attacks compared to those not taking calcium.[328]

Osteoporosis is due to poor nutrition, chemicals, and lack of physical activity. So the first thing to do is to eat Paleo, be active, and avoid chemicals whenever possible. The best source of calcium is from food such as vegetables and small fish such as anchovy, sardines, and herring. Bone broth made from free-range animals is packed with vitamins and minerals, including calcium along with the ever-important saturated fat. Get some grass-fed cow bones and put them in a large pot of water. Boiling for 24-48 hours will soften them and you will be able to drink all of the nutrients. You can use the broth as stock for other soups or consume on its own.

The second best thing you can do is take The Drs. Wolfson MULTI, which contains the vitamins necessary for bone health. Our MULTI contains vitamin C, D, K, magnesium, boron, and a small amount of calcium along with all of the other vitamins for outstanding health. Digestive enzymes and betaine HCL are also important supplements for those looking to keep their bones strong.

ACTION PLAN

1. Vitamins, minerals, and supplements are proven to work. The science is there.
2. Make sure you take top quality supplements. You can trust TheDrsWolfson.com for the finest products available.
3. Check with your doctor to see which supplements are appropriate for you.
4. Read the next chapter for the tests you need to determine your supplement requirements.

Chapter 17

TOP TWENTY BLOOD TESTS

"One-quarter of what you eat keeps you alive.
The other three-quarters keeps your doctor alive."
—*Egyptian Proverb*

There are many different tests to determine cardiac risk. Many tests are very useful to determine the cause of just about every symptom or health problem that exists. If your doctor is not checking these, find one who does. Here are my Top 20 tests, many of which are covered by insurance. Check with your carrier first.

1. **Advanced lipid analysis**—Instead of the 1970's test of total cholesterol, LDL, HDL, and triglycerides, this really looks under the hood, so to speak. In this test, HDL and LDL particle numbers and size are determined. These are much more predictive of risk than the old test. This test also checks the nasty LDL called Lp(a). It is very important

to know if this number is high as it is a leading cause of familial heart disease.

2. **Diabetes panel**—this group includes tests such as fasting glucose, insulin, and the three-month control of sugar, Hgb A1C. Fructosamine, adiponectin, and leptin also provide metabolic information.

3. **Homocysteine**—a protein linked with an increased risk of heart attacks, strokes, blood clots, cancer, dementia, and death. Knowing your blood level is critical.

4. **Inflammation markers**—hs-CRP, PLA2, IL1b, TNF, IL-6. The more inflammation, the higher the risk of disease. CRP raises blood pressure and causes vasoconstriction. It is a marker of disease and contributes to worsening hypertension, and blockages.

5. **Oxidation markers**—lipid peroxides, myeloperoxidase and F2 isoprostanes. If these are high, the body is suffering extreme damage. If you really want to know your risk of heart and other diseases, ask for these markers.

6. **Food sensitivity panel**—Quite simply, do you react negatively to certain foods and could these foods be leading to disease? If so, avoid them. When the results are abnormal, there is definitely a problem. But if your test is normal for a food, it does not mean you are out of the woods. For example, one test may not reveal a gluten problem, but more extensive tests may uncover it as an issue. One of the best tests is a question: How do you feel after eating a particular food? Monitor for symptoms up to 48 hours later.

7. **Heavy metals**—whether by blood, urine, or hair, find out your metal burden.

8. **Genetics**—MTHFR, Factor V Leiden, Apo E, Prothrombin gene mutation, and KIF 6. This list is growing every day and there can be plenty of confusion. Nonetheless, it pays to know your DNA. Several websites allow you to plug in your DNA from 23andMe.com and get information. Do it.

9. **Thyroid**—Numbers here are very important and there is a tight range of normalcy. Autoimmune markers, such as anti-thyroglobulin and anti-

thyroid peroxidase, are very important. Elevation in one or both of these antibodies lets us know something (poor nutrition and chemicals) is attacking your thyroid and likely other parts of your body.

10. **Genova Diagnostics**—This company offers panels with incredible information from blood, urine, and stool. Gut function, metals, intracellular nutrients, protein and carbohydrate metabolism, lipid peroxides, etc. are just a few of the tests which are of critical value in determining your health status.

11. **Vitamin D**—This hormone is responsible for many bodily functions, and every disease is more common in those people with low levels. You need to know.

12. **Leaky Gut**—Cyrex is a company based out of Phoenix with a unique test for intestinal permeability. If your gut is leaky, you had better find out the cause and fix it fast.

13. **Infections**—Whether by blood or stool analysis, the bugs must be found. Bacterial overgrowth, yeast, and parasites can wreak havoc on your body and need to be eradicated. Stool testing can also be used to assess your digestive capabilities and need for digestive enzyme therapy.

14. **Spectracell**—This company offers a test to look at intracellular nutrients AND vitamins along with CoQ10 level and anti-oxidant status. If you are taking plenty of supplements, wouldn't you like to know if they are working?

15. **Omega 3 Index**—Do your cells contain enough omega 3 fats in their membranes? The lower your index, the higher your cardiovascular risk. Omega 3 fatty acids in the cell membrane help cells "talk" with each other and other molecules (such as hormones) circulating in the body. If levels are low, eat wild salmon and anchovies to boost, and take an omega 3 DHA/EPA supplement.

16. **Neurotransmitters**—Usually performed by saliva testing: dopamine, norepinephrine, GABA, and serotonin levels are very useful in patients with conditions from anxiety and panic to hypertension and heart rhythm problems.

17. **Adrenal function**—Another saliva test to assess cortisol levels four times throughout the day. Low cortisol can lead to many symptoms such as fatigue, lightheadedness, and sleep problems. This list goes on. Labrix is my choice here.

18. **Sex hormones**—Finding a proper balance with male and female hormones is very important. Bio-identical replacement can be tricky and does not go after the CAUSE of the problem. Very often, hormone replacement is not necessary when the diet is cleaned up and the toxins are removed.

19. **Galectin-3 and BNP**—Are very useful to determine heart stress. If levels are high, the cause needs to be found. Usually this is a sign blood pressure is elevated, or the heart function is not normal. Leaky heart valves can also lead to a rise in heart stress.

20. **Uric acid**—Another risk marker when elevated. The cause of the elevation is sugar and starchy carbs. High uric acid leads to painful arthritic symptoms named gout. High uric acid is a risk factor for heart disease.

ACTION PLAN:

1. Do not settle for basic, 1970's blood tests.
2. Blood, saliva, urine and other noninvasive tests provide great information.
3. Skip the tests that subject you to unnecessary radiation.
4. You and your health team should come up with a plan based on your history and bloodtest results.
5. Repeat these tests as necessary to ensure you are constantly tracking your results.

AFTERWORD

I realize your head is likely spinning from all of the information in this book. Don't panic, and remember, slow and steady wins the race. Although many of my patients are able to embrace these recommendations very quickly, others need time. It is very understandable given the fact the vast majority of your life was likely similar to mine, where fast food and Tide laundry detergent were the norm. You cannot learn another language in a day. Years of practice are necessary. Changing your nutrition and lifestyle is a continuous evolution. But the rewards will be longevity and vitality. We want to thrive, not just survive.

No matter your medical history, it is never too late to change. Whether you have had bypass surgery, stents, a heart attack, or an ablation, your health can dramatically improve. One day at a time, you can heal yourself. For years, I have saved patients from useless pills and procedures. You can be one of those patients.

The journey to health has many detours and diversions. We all succumb to poor choices when under stress or when bad things happen. Sometimes, it's just a birthday or holiday that throws us off track. But the important thing is not to give up. Just wake up the next day and make it a good food day. Pick a date to resume your healthy lifestyle. Take a week off work and start a juice fast. Clear out all of the unhealthy food from the house. If you do not make the time to prevent and heal disease, your health will suffer.

Create a natural health care team. Find a general doc, chiropractor, and dentist who think holistically. Bear in mind, many of these doctors will not accept insurance. The best never do. Insurance limits the care a doctor can provide. Office visits are short and the best tests may not be "covered." Insurance companies, pharmaceutical companies, and the government do not care about us. They care about profit and they are all in a nice, cozy bed together. It is time for us to throw an ice bucket on that arrangement.

Never mind the naysayers. Give them a copy of *The Paleo Cardiologist*. Teach others what you learned, for this is the greatest gift you could ever give. My wife gave it to me and now I give it to you. But if those in your life refuse to change or impede your progress, sometimes you must make tough decisions. Nonetheless, do not allow yourself to be held back from optimum health and wellness.

The Drs. Wolfson are here to guide you. Please continue to watch what we are doing. Read our posts, watch our videos, and listen to our lectures. Heed our advice on holistic living and healthy nutrition. Let us do the research. Most importantly, just do what makes common sense: If not for yourself, for future generations.

Please find us at TheDrsWolfson.com and all social media under TheDrsWolfson.

Help us change the world.

Thank you.

ABOUT THE AUTHOR

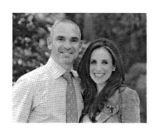 Dr. Jack Wolfson was born in Cleveland, Ohio. His father was the first osteopathic physician at the Cleveland Clinic. The family moved to Chicago where Dr. Wolfson was raised and did all of his training. He received his B.S. in Biology from The University of Illinois with dreams of following in his father's footsteps. He then enrolled at Midwestern University for his medical school training. He did a subsequent three-year residency in Internal Medicine and three year fellowship in Cardiology. In his final year, Dr. Wolfson was appointed Chief Fellow.

After finishing his training, Dr. Wolfson moved to Arizona in 2002. He joined a large cardiology group and was elected as a senior partner in 2006. After years of angiograms, pacemakers, and other procedures, Dr. Wolfson met the woman who opened his eyes to the wellness paradigm. Dr. Jack and Dr. Heather now practice as The Drs. Wolfson.

In 2012, Dr. Wolfson opened his own private practice with the idea of providing patients in-depth information about their health and the risks and benefits of all treatments. The focus is to use nutrition, evidence-based supplements, chemical avoidance, exercise, and relaxation to prevent and treat cardiovascular disease. Patients seek his consultation from all over the world.

The Drs. Wolfson have two beautiful boys and live in Arizona. They have a rescue lab-mix named Sal. They love to hike and bike as a family. They are active soccer parents. The family eats organic food, grass-fed meats, and wild seafood. Both boys were born at home and breastfed for over three years. The Drs. Wolfson practice attachment parenting and co-sleep with their boys.

END NOTES

CHAPTER 1

1   Chu LW <u>J Alzheimer's Dis</u>. 2010; 21(4):1335-45. Bioavailable testosterone predicts a lower risk of Alzheimer's disease in older men.

2   Rosano GM <u>Int J Impot Res</u>. 2007 Mar-Apr; 19(2):176-82. Low testosterone levels are associated with coronary artery disease in male patients with angina.

3   J. Clin Endocrinol Metab. 2010 Nov: 95 (11): 4985-92

4   Cancer Lett. 1979 Sep: 7 (5): 273-82.

5   For more information visit, Spectracell.com

6   <u>J Clin Neurosci.</u> 2014 Jul 28.

7   West R. <u>Am J Geriatr Psychiatry</u>. 2008 Sep;16(9):781-5

8   Vilibic M. <u>Croat Med J</u>. 2014 Oct 30;55(5):520-9.

CHAPTER 2

9   <u>J Gerontol A Biol Sci Med Sci.</u> 2008 Feb;63(2):122-6.

10   Toth PP. Reverse cholesterol transport: High-density lipoprotein's magnificent mile. Curr Atheroscler Rep. 2003;5:386-93.

11   American Journal of Medicine, 1977;62;707-714

12   Toth PP. Reverse cholesterol transport: High-density lipoprotein's magnificent mile. Curr Atheroscler Rep. 2003;5:386-93.

13   American Journal of Medicine, 1977;62;707-714

14   Circulation. 2007; 115: 450-458

15   Circulation. 2008 Jan 15;117(2):176-84.

16   Arteriosclerosis, Thrombosis, and Vascular Biology 1997; 17:1657-61.

CHAPTER 3

17   Diabetologia. 2007 Sep; 50(9):1795-807.

18   PREDIMED Primary Prevention of Cardiovascular Disease with a Mediterranean Diet. N Engl J Med 2013; 368:1279-1290.

19   Beneficial Effects of a Paleo Diet versus a Diabetes Diet: A randomized cross-over trial. Cardiovasc Diabetol. 2009; 8: 35.

20   Diabetes. 1984 Jun;33(6):596-603.

21   BMJ. Sep 28, 1996; 313(7060): 775–779.

22   The FASEB Journal. 2007;21:769.20.

23   Am J Clin Nutr April 1988 vol. 47 no. 4 660-663.

24   J Steroid Biochem. 1989 Jun;32(6):829-33

25   Am J Clin Nutr January 1999vol. 69 no. 1 147-152

26   Asia Pac J Clin Nutr. 2006;15(1):21-9.

27   Nutr J. 2010 Mar 10;9:10

28   http://ec.europa.eu/food/fs/sc/scv/out19_en.html

29   Epidemiology: January 2011 - Volume 22 - Issue 1 - pp S107-S108

30   Mozaffarian D JAMA. 2006; 296:1885-99.1.

31   Pischon T. Circulation.2003;108:155-60; van Bussel BC. J Nutr. 2011;141:1719-25.

32   Nutr J. 2014 Jan 9;13(1).

33   Int J Endocrinol. 2013; 2013: 501015

34   Ann Nutr Metab. 2008;52(1):37-47.

35   J Am Coll Nutr. 2011 Dec;30(6):502-10.

36   Nutrients. 2010 Jul;2(7):652-82.

37   NEJM. 369:2001-2011.

38   British Journal of Nutrition / Volume 111 / Issue 12 / June 2014, pp 2146-2152.

39   JAMA. 2008 August 27; 300(8): 907=914.

40   J Nutr. 2008 Feb;138(2):272-6.

41   British Journal of Nutrition / Volume 112 / Issue 10 / November 2014, pp 1636-1643.

42   Crit Rev Food Sci Nutr. May 2013; 53(7): 738–750.

43   Crit Rev Food Sci Nutr. 2013 May; 53(7): 738-750.

44   Chemotherapy. 2013;59(3):214-24.

45   Am J Clin Nutr. 2003 May;77(5):1146-55.

46   Southeast Asian J Trop Med Public Health. 2012 Jul;43(4):969-85.

47   Asia Pac J Clin Nutr. 2011;20(2):190-5.

48   J Nutr Biochem. 2014 Feb;25(2):144-50.

49   Phytother Res. 2013 Aug 7.

50   Nutr Biochem. 2008 June; 19(6): 347-361.

CHAPTER 4

51   Bang and Dyerberg: Advances in Nutrition Research 1980:1-22.

52   Siri-Tarino: Amer J of Clin Nutr. Jan 13, 2010.

53   JAMA Intern Med. Published online February 03, 2014.

54   Diabetes Care June 2008 vol. 31 no. 6 1144-1149.

55   Rev Esp Cardiol. 2009;62(05):528.

56   JAMA.2002;288(21):2709-2716.

57   Cardiac manifestations of acute carbamate and organophosphate poisoning. A.M. Saadeh. Heart. May 1997; 77(5): 461-464.

58   Circulating Levels of Persistent Organic Pollutants (POPs) and Carotid Atherosclerosis in the Elderly. P Monica Lind. Environ Health Perspect. Jan 2012; 120(1): 38-43.

59   Seneff S. Entropy 2013, 15, 1416-1463.

60   http://www.beyondpesticides.org/health/pid-database.pdf.

61   Br J Nutr. Sep 14, 2014; 112(5): 794–811.

62   Fowler, S.P. Obesity 2008:16, 1894-1900.

63   Fagerrazzi. Amer Journ Clin Nutr 2013:97, 517-523.

64   Fung. AJCN 2009: 89,1037.

65   Int Journ of Cardiology; Volume 137, Issue 3. 307-308.

66   Anal Bioanal Chem 2012 Jul, 403(9): 2503-18.

67   Pak J Biol Sci. 2012 Oct 1;15(19):904-18.

68   Amer J Physiol Heart Circ Physiol. 2003;284:1184; Autonomic
      Neuroscience 2003;105:105;
      Am J Physiol Regul Integ Comp Physiol 2001;281:R935; Eur J
      Pharmacol 1994;252:155; J Nutr Sci Vitaminol (Tokyo) 2003;49:145.

CHAPTER 5

69   https://www.apa.org/news/press/releases/stress/2011/final-2011.pdf

70   Curr Opin Psychiatry. 2015 Jan;28(1):1-6.

71   Gut Microbes. 2013 Jan-Feb;4(1):17-27.

72   Haley et al. Stroke. 2010;41:331-36.

73   Psychosomatic Medicine:April 2014 - Volume 76 - Issue 3 - p 181-189.

74   Milani R., Lavie CJ. Postgrad Med. 2011 Sep;123(5):165-76.

75   JAMA Intern Med. 2014;174(4):598-605.

76   De Bacquer. Am J Epidemiol 2005;161:434-441.

77   Castillo-Richmond Stroke 2000; 31:568-573.

78   Psychosomatic Medicine: November/December 2013 - Volume 75 -
      Issue 9.

79   Clin Res Cardiol. 2013 Nov;102(11):807-11.

80   Everson SA. Arterioscler Thromb Vasc Biol 1997 Aug;17(8):1490-5).

81   Vidovich Cardiovascular Psychiatry and Neurology Volume 2009.

82   J Psychosom Res. 2007 Nov;63(5):509-13.

83   BMJ. 1987;295:297-299.

84   Circulation. 1994;89:1992-1997.

85   Circulation.1994;90:2225-2229.

86   Circulation. 1996;94:2090-2095.

87   J Am Coll Cardiol. 2011 Sep 13;58(12):1222-8.

88   European Journal of Preventive Cardiology. Jan 30, 2013.

89   Gen Hosp Psychiatry. 2014 Mar-Apr;36(2):142-9.

90   Heart Lung Circ. 2013 Apr;22(4):291-6.

91   Circulation. 2004 Mar 16;109(10):1267-71.

92   Stroke.1993;24:983-986.

93   Mayo Clin Proc. 1996;71:729-734.

94   Psychosom Med. 2001 Mar-Apr;63(2):267-72.

95   Soc Sci Med. May 2011; 72(9): 1482-1488.

CHAPTER 6

96   Annual Review of Public Health. Vol. 33: 157-68.

97   www.cdc.gov/medicationsafety/adult_adversedrugevents.html

98   BMJ Open. April 8, 2014.

99   JAMA 1998; 279:1615-1622.

100   N Engl J Med 1995; 333:1301-1308.

101   N Engl J Med 2008; 359:2195-2207

102   Lancet 1994; 344:1383-1389

103   JAMA. 2014;311(5):507-520.

104   BMJ 2011;342:d2234.

105   Lancet. 1997; 350:757-764

106   J Renin Angiotensin Aldosterone Syst. 2002 Jun;3(2):61-2.

107   Lancet Oncol. 2010 Jul;11(7):627-36).

108   N Engl J Med 2000; 342:145-153

109   JAMA Intern Med. 2014;174(4):588-595

110   Cancer Epidemiol Biomarkers Prev. Published Online First May 15,
      2014.

111   Am J Gastroenterol 2005;100:1685-93

112   Br J Clin Pharmacol. Mar 2003; 55(3): 282-287.

113   Arthritis Rheum. 2000 Jan;43(1):103-8.

114   Isr Med Assoc J. 2006 Oct;8(10):679-82.

115   JAMA Intern Med. 2013;173(4):258-264

116   Am Surg. 2014 Oct;80(10):920-5.

117   Acta Otorhinolaryngol Ital. 2014 Apr;34(2):79-93.

118   N Engl J Med. 2014 Dec 4;371(23):2155-66.

119   CAST Trial N Engl J Med.1989;321:406-412

120   NEJM 2008; 358: 2545-59

121   https://circ.ahajournals.org/content/100/25/e133.full

122   NEJM 2010; 362:1575-8.

123   JAMA. 1998 Apr 15;279(15):1200-5.

CHAPTER 7

124   *JAMA.* 2014;311(13):1327-1335.

125   JAMA Internal Medicine: Feb 10, 2014

126   circ.ahajournals.org/content/130/Suppl_2/A16701.short.

127   Scientific American Volume 309, Issue 1.

128   Circ Cardiovasc Interv. 2014;7:19-27

129   N Engl J Med 2007; 356:1503-1516

130   Journal of the American College of Cardiology Volume 16, Issue 5, 1
      November 1990, Pages 1071-078

131   N Engl J Med 2011; 364:1607-1616

132   Bardy G.H. Sudden Cardiac Death in Heart Failure Trial (SCD-HeFT)
      Investigators Amiodarone or an implantable cardioverter-defibrillator for
      congestive heart failure. N Engl J Med. 352 2005:225-237.

133   Peters A, et al. Air pollution and incidence of cardiac
      arrhythmia. Epidemiology. 2000;11:11-7; Baccarelli A, , et al. Exposure
      to particulate air pollution and risk of deep vein thrombosis. Arch Intern
      Med. 2008;168:920-7.

CHAPTER 8

134   Lim SS. A comparative risk assessment of burden of disease and injury
      attributable to 67 risk factor clusters in 21 regions, 1990-2010: a
      systematic analysis for the Global Burden of Disease Study 2010. Lancet
      2012;380:2224-60

135   Cesaroni, G. BMJ 2014;348:f7412 doi: 10.1136/bmj.f7412

136   Raaschou-Nielsen, O. Environmental Health. September 2012, 11:60

137   Brook RD, et al. Air pollution and cardiovascular disease.
      Circulation. 2002;109:2655-71; Holguín F, et al. Air pollution

and heart rate variability among the elderly in Mexico City. Epidemiology. 2003;14:521-7.

138   Lhoret. JCEM. Feb 25, 2014.

139   NEJM. 2007 Sep 13; 357(11):1075-82.

140   Eur Heart J. 2011 Nov;32(21):2660-71.

141   Arch Environ Health 1981;36(2):59-66.

142   Am J Epidemiol 1988 Dec;128(6):1276-1288.

143   PLoS Comput Biol 10(3): e1003518.

144   I recommend Austin out of Buffalo.

145   http://www.cdc.gov/tobacco/data_statistics/fact_sheets/secondhand_smoke/health_effects/

146   J Am Coll Cardiol Img 2013;651-657.

147   Cardiol J. 2008;15(4):338-43.

148   http://www.plosone.org/article/info%3Adoi%2F10.1371%2Fjournal.pone.0086391

149   Ehrlich S, et al. JAMA. Feb 26, 2014. 859-860.

150   Melzer D, et al. (2012) Urinary Bisphenol A Concentration and Angiography-Defined Coronary Artery Stenosis. PLoS ONE 7(8): e43378. doi:10.1371/journal.pone.0043378

151   Effects of electromagnetic field exposure on the heart: a systematic review. Onur Elmas Toxicol Ind Health 10 September 2013.

152   Arch Intern Med. 2012;172(18):1397-1403.

153   Diabetologia. 2014 Mar;57(3):473-9.

154   Diabetologia. 2014 Mar;57(3):473-9.

155   Toxicol Res. 2012 Dec;28(4):269-77.

156   SJWEH Suppl 2006;(2):54-60.

157   South Med J. 1980 Aug;73(8):1081-3.

158   Toxicol Appl Pharmacol. 2013 Apr 15;268(2):157-77.

CHAPTER 9

159   Bhatnagar A. Environmental cardiology: studying mechanistic links between pollution and heart disease. Circulation Research. 2006;99(7):692–705.

160 Alissa E. J Toxicol. 2011.

161 Staessen JA. Hypertension caused by low-level lead exposure: myth or fact? Journal of Cardiovascular Risk. 1994;1(1):87–97

162 Am J Ind Med. 1988;13(6):659-66; Costello S. Incident ischemic heart disease and recent occupational exposure to particulate matter in an aluminum cohort. J Expo Sci Environ Epidemiol. 2014 Jan-Feb;24(1):82-8.

163 Am J Ind Med. 1988;13(6):659-66; Schwartz J. Lead, blood pressure, and cardiovascular disease in men. Archives of Environmental Health. 1995;50; (1):31–37; Nawrot TS An epidemiological re-appraisal of the association between blood pressure and blood lead: a meta-analysis. Journal of Human Hypertension.2002;16(2):123–131.

164 Costello, S. Incident ischemic heart disease and recent occupational exposure to particulate matter in an aluminum cohort. J Expo Sci Environ Epidemiol. 2014 Jan-Feb;24(1):82-8.

165 Am J Epidemiol. Feb 2009; 169(4): 489-496.

166 Am J Epidemiol. Feb 2009; 169(4): 489–496; Simeonova PP, Luster MI. Arsenic and atherosclerosis. Toxicology and Applied Pharmacology.2004;198:444–449.

167 Wang CH, et al. Circulation. 2002;105:1804–1809; Chiou HY. Stroke. 1997;28(9):1717–1723.

168 Tseng CH, et al. Long-term arsenic exposure and ischemic heart disease in arseniasis-hyperendemic villages in Taiwan. Toxicology Letters. 2003;137(1-2):15–21.

169 Gallagher CM. Blood and urine cadmium, blood pressure, and hypertension: a systematic review and meta-analysis. Environmental Health Perspectives. 2010;118(12):1676–1684; Haswell-Elkins M. Striking association between urinary cadmium level and albuminuria among Torres Strait Islander people with diabetes. Environmental Research 2008;106(3):379–383; Schwartz GG. Urinary cadmium, impaired fasting glucose, and diabetes in the NHANES III. Diabetes Care. 2003;26(2):468–470.

170   Houtman JP. Prolonged low-level cadmium intake and atherosclerosis. Science of the Total Environment. 1993;138(1–3):31–36.

171   J Toxicol Sci. 2011 Jan;36(1):121-6; Nutr Res Pract. 2009 Summer;3(2):89-94

172   JAMA. Mar 27, 2013; 309(12): 1241–1250.

CHAPTER 10
173   NEJM. 2008; 359: 2195-2207.

174   The Lancet, Volume 375, Issue 9725, Pages 1536 - 1544, 1 May 2010.

175   European Heart Journal (2006) 27, 2346-2352.

176   Am. Heart J. 163 (4): 666-76.

177   Holvoet, P, et al. Diabetes, April 2004; 1068-73.

178   Cardiovasc Diagn Ther. 2012 December; 2(4): 298-307.

179   Heart 2011;97:1636-42.

180   BMC Cardiovasc Disord. 2014 Apr 16;14:52.

181   Circ Arrhythm Electrophysiol. 2012 Apr;5(2):327-33.

182   Indian J Biochem Biophys. 2009 Dec;46(6):498-502.

183   Rose, GA ; 1531-33. BMJ 1965

184   J Biol Regul Homeost Agents. 2012 Jan-Mar;26(1 Suppl):S63-8.

CHAPTER 11
185   BMC Genomics. 2013 May 30;14:362.

186   SLEEP 2011;34(11):1487-1492.

187   Am J Cardiol. 2013 Mar 1;111(5):631-5.

188   Am J Hypertens. 2013 Jul;26(7):903-11. Hypertension. 2006 May;47(5):833-9.

189   Yigiang Zhan. Sleep Medicine Volume 15, Issue 7, Pages 833–839, July 2014

190   Physiol Behav. 2010 Dec 2;101(5):693-8

191   Journal of Sleep Research. 2011;20:298.

192   Neurobiology of Aging, 2014.

193   World J Gastroenterol. 2013 Dec 28;19(48):9231-9.

194 PLoS One. 2014 Apr 3;9(4):e91965.

195 China Medical University in Taiwan.

196 J Adolesc Health. 2012 Dec;51(6):615-22.

197 J Clin Oncol. 2013 Sep 10;31(26):3233-41; J Bodyw Mov Ther. 2013 Jan;17(1):5-10.

CHAPTER 12

198 Physical activity, all-cause mortality, and longevity of college alumni. Paffenbarger RS Jr et al. N Engl J Med 1986;314:605-13.

199 Leisure-time running reduces all-cause and cardiovascular mortality risk. Duck-chul Lee, PhD et al. JACC. 2014; 64(5):472.

200 Cardiac rehabilitation after myocardial infarction: Combined experience of randomized clinical trials. Oldridge NB et al. JAMA 1988;260:945-50.

201 Relationship between Physical Activity and Plasma Fibrinogen Concentrations in Adults without Chronic Diseases. Gomez-Marcos et al. PLoS One. 2014 Feb 3;9(2):e8795.

202 Acute and chronic effects of exercise on inflammatory markers and B-type natriuretic peptide in patients with coronary artery disease. Fernandes L. et al. Clin Res Cardiol. 2011 Jan;100(1):77-84.

203 Sinus node and arrhythmias in the long term follow up of professional cyclists. Baldesberger S. et al. Eur Heart J (2008) 29 (1): 71-78.

204 Effects of yoga on cardiovascular disease risk factors: a systematic review and meta-analysis. Cramer H. Int J Cardiol. 2014 Feb 25.

205 Impact of yoga on arrhythmia burden. Lakkireddy. JACC. 2011; 57: E129.

206 Chuang et al. Spine. 37 (18): 1593-160. See also http://en.wikipedia.org/wiki/Yoga - cite_note-pmid22433499-218.

207 Yoga for Chronic Low Back Pain in a Predominantly Minority Population: A Pilot Randomized Controlled Trial. Dugan et al. Alternative Therapies. November 2009.

208 BMC Public Health. 2004 Nov 30;4:56.

CHAPTER 13

209 J Med Food. 2012 Jun;15(6):535-41.

210 Am J Epidemiol. 1988 Sep;128(3):570-8.

211 Am J Epidemiol. 1990 Sep;132(3):479-88.

212 Mayo Clinic Proceedings October 2013.

213 Am J Clin Nutr. 2011 Oct;94(4):1113-26.

214 Circ Res. 2010 Mar 5;106(4):779-87.

215 Biochemistry (Mosc). 2004 Jan;69(1):70-4.

216 J Toxicol. 2013;2013:370460.

217 Stroke. 2014 Jan;45(1):309-14.

218 Cochrane Database Syst Rev. 2013 Jun 18;6.

219 Am J Clin Nutr. 2013 Dec;98.

220 Fitoterapia. 2011 Apr;82(3):309-16.

221 Stroke 2013; 44: 1369-74.

222 Mayo Clin Proc. 2014 Mar;89(3):382-93

223 Mayo Clin Proc. 2014 Mar;89(3):382-93.

224 *JAMA*. 2004 Aug 25;292(8):927-34.

225 J Sch Nurs. 2008 Feb;24(1):3-12.

226 Future Cardiol. 2010 Nov;6(6):773-6.

227 Cancer Epidemiol Biomarkers Prev. 2005 Sep;14(9):2098-105.

228 http://www.prevention.com/food/healthy-eating-tips/soda-and-endometrial-cancer.

229 Am J Clin Nutr. 2006 Oct;84(4):936-42.

230 http://www.cancer.gov/cancertopics/factsheet/Risk/formaldehyde.

231 Diabetes Care April 2009 vol. 32 no. 4 688-694.

232 http://www.cardiosource.org/en/News-Media/Media-Center/News-Releases/2014/03/Vyas-Diet-Drinks.aspx

233 Eur J Nutr. 2014 Jan 29.

234 Ebina S. Int J Womens Health. 2012; 4: 333–339.

CHAPTER 14

235 Kleiger R. Amer Jour of Cardio. Feb 1, 1987. Vol 59:4. Pg 256–262

236 Brennan PC, et al. JMPT, 1991;14:399-408.

237 J Chiropr Med. 2011 Mar;10(1):60-3.

238 J Hum Hypertens. 2007 May; 21(5): 347-52

239 J Altern Complement Med. 2011 Sep;17(9):797-801.

240 - J Chiropr Med. 2008 Sep;7(3):86-93.

241 J Manipulative Physiol Ther. 2009 May;32(4):277-86; J Manipulative Physiol Ther. 2006 May;29(4):267-74.

242 J Chiropr Med. 2010 Sep;9(3):107-14.

243 J Manipulative Physiol Ther. 2012 Jan;35(1):7-17.

CHAPTER 15

244 Caplan DJ. ; J Dent Res. Nov 2006; 85(11): 996–1000.Elter JR.J Periodontol. 2004 Jun;75(6):782-90.

245 Colomb Med (Cali). 2013 Jun 30;44(2):80-6.

246 Frisbee. J Dent Hyg. 2010 Fall;84(4):177-84.

247 Caplan DJ. J Am Dent Assoc. 2009 Aug;140(8):1004-12.

248 Gundry, SR et al "Teeth Flossing Habits Directly Correlate with Serum hs C-Reactive Protein Levels: Plaque in the Mouth-Plaque in the Arteries" Poster 232.

CHAPTER 16

249 Journal of the American College of Nutrition. Volume 32, Issue 5, 2013.

250 Human Psychopharmacology. Vol 25, Issue 6, 448-461, August 2010.

251 JAMA. November 14, 2012, Vol 308, No. 18.

252 Br J Nutr. 2013 Nov 14;110(9):1685-95.

253 J Am Coll Nutr. 2011 Feb;30(1):49-56.

254 http://wolfsonintegrativecardiology.com/8-ways-chlorella-benefits-body/ - ref14,

255 http://wolfsonintegrativecardiology.com/8-ways-chlorella-benefits-body/ - ref13.

256 http://wolfsonintegrativecardiology.com/8-ways-chlorella-benefits-body.

257 http://wolfsonintegrativecardiology.com/amazing-health-benefits-spirulina/

258 J Cardiovasc Pharmacol. 2014 Jul;64(1):87-99.

259   Am J Clin Nutr 2013, 2, 268-75.

260   Eur J Pharmacol. 2013 Jul 5;711(1-3):1-9.

261   PLoS One. 2012; 7(8): e43229.

262   J Nutr. 2004;134:3100-310; Atherosclerosis. 2009;203:489-493; Nutr Metab Cardiovasc Dis. 2009;19:504-510.

263   Thromb Haemost. 2004;91:373-80.

264   Am J Epidemiol. Feb 1, 2008; 167(3) 313-320.

265   Diabetes Care September 2011vol. 34 no. 9 e147.

266   Am J Clin Nutr April 2008 vol. 87no. 4 985-992.

267   J Nutr. 2014 Mar 19.

268   U Md Med Cntr. May 7, 20132.

269   Hypertension. 2014 Mar;63(3):459-673.

270   Free Radical Biology and Medicine 51(5): 1000-13.

271   Proc Natl Acad Sci U S A. 92(18): 8171-8175.

272   Gerontology. 2012;58(1):62-9.

273   Free Radical Biology and Medicine. Oct. 23, 2000.

274   J Am Coll Cardiol. 2013 Oct 15;62(16):1457-65.

275   JAMA. 2014 Jan 1;311(1):33-44.

276   Am J Clin Nutr. 2014 Jan;99(1):107-14.

277   Sato K. Arzneimittelforschung.2006;56:535–540.

278   Simon JA. J Am Coll Nutr. 1992 Apr;11(2):107-25.

279   Tex Heart Inst J. 2007;34(3):268-74.

280   Asher A. et al. Atherosclerosis. July 2014.

281   Pfeifer M. J Clin Endocrinol Metab. 2001;86:1633–1637.

282   Birdsall T, Kelly G. Berberine: therapeutic potential of an alkaloid in several medicinal plants. Alt Med Rev. 1997;2(2):94-103.

283   Srivastava RA. J Lipid Res. 2012;53(12):2490-2514.

284   Jeong HW. Am J Physiol Endocrinol Metab. 2009;296 (4):E955-964;

285   Dong H. Berberine in the treatment of type 2 diabetes mellitus. Evid Based Complement Alternat Med. 2012;2012:591654.

286   Kong W. Berberine is a novel cholesterol-lowering drug working through a unique mechanism distinct from statins. Nat Med. 2004;10(12):1344-1351.

287   Guan S, Wang B, Li W, Guan J, Fang X. Effects of berberine on expression of LOX-1 and SR-BI in human macrophage-derived foam cells induced by ox-LDL. Am J Chin Med. 2010;38 (6):1161-1169.

288   Xie X. *Zhongguo Zhong Yao Za Zhi*.2011;36(21):3032-3035.

289   Zhang H. Berberine lowers blood glucose in type 2 diabetes mellitus patients through increasing insulin receptor expression. Metabolism. 2010;59(2):285-292.

290   Wang Y. Berberine and plant stanols synergistically inhibit cholesterol absorption. Atherosclerosis. 2010;209 (1):111-117.

291   Kong WJ, Wei J, Zuo ZY, et al. Combination of simvastatin with berberine improves the lipid-lowering efficacy. Metabolism. 2008;57(8):1029-1037.

292   Ko WH, Yao XQ, Lau CW, et al. Vasorelaxant and antiproliferative effects of berberine. Eur J Pharmacol.2000;399(2-3):187-196.

293   Zeng XH, Zeng XJ, Li YY. Efficacy and safety of berberine for congestive heart failure secondary to ischemic or idiopathic dilated cardiomyopathy. Am J Cardiol. 2003;92 (2):173-176.

294   Check out Alternative Medicine Review Volume 15, Number 2 for more information.

295   Oral L-citrulline supplementation improves erection hardness in men with mild erectile dysfunction. Cormio L, et al. Urology. 2011 Jan;77(1):119-22.

296   Improvement of ventricular function in systolic heart failure patients with oral L-citrulline supplementation. Balderas-Munoz K. Cardiol J. 2012;19(6):612-7.

297   The effect of L-arginine and citrulline on endothelial function in patients in heart failure with preserved ejection fraction. Orea A. Cardiol J. 2010; 17(5) :464-70.

298   Citrulline/malate promotes aerobic energy production in human exercising muscle. Bendahan D. Br J Sports Med 2002;36:282-289.

299   soils.wisc.edu/facstaff/barak/poster_gallery/minneapolis2000a.

300   Archives of Med Res. 2014 Jul;45(5):388-93.

301   Archives of Med Res. 2014 Jul;45(5):388-93.

302   Archives of Med Res. 2014 Jul;45(5):388-93.

303   Arch of Med Res.2014 May 325-30.

304   Diabetes Med. 2006 Oct;23(10):1050-6.

305   International Journal of Cardiology 179 (2015) 348–350.

306   Amino Acids. 2002; WJC 2013.

307   Amino Acids 26 (3): 267-71.

308   Life Sci.2002;70:2355-2366.

309   Jpn Circ J.1992 Jan;56(1):95-9.

310   Clin Cardiol. 1985 May;8(5):276-82.

311   J Cardiol. 2011 May;57(3):333-7.

312   Diab Vasc Dis Res. 2010 Oct;7(4):300-10.

313   Amino Acids 26 (2): 203-7.

314   Eby G. Med Hypotheses. 2006;67(5):1200-4.

315   Garlic: A review of potential therapeutic effects. Bayan L. et al. Avicenna J Phytomed. 2014. Jan-Feb; 1-14.

316   J Nutr. 2013 Jun;143(6):818-26.

317   My clinical experience. No data found.

318   Atherosclerosis. 2013 Nov;231(1):78-83.

319   Med Sci Sports Exerc. 2014 Jan;46(1):143-50.

320   Free Radic Biol Med. 2013 Jul;60:89-97.

321   J Appl Physiol 2011 Jun;110(6):1582-91.

322   Plant Foods Hum Nutr. 2010 Jun;65(2):105-11.

323   Hypertension. 2008;51(3):784–790.

324   Sumi. Acta Haematol 1990;84(3):139-43.

325   Jang JY. Lab Anim Res. 2013 Dec;29(4):221-5.

326   Fadl NN. Hum Exp Toxicol. 2013 Jul;32(7):721-35.

327   Cicero AF. Nutr Res. 2013 Aug;33(8):622-8; Lee CY. Forsch Komplementmed. 2013;20(3):197-203; Halbert SC. Am J Cardiol. 2010 Jan 15;105(2):198-204; Liu L. Clin Chem. 2003 Aug;49(8):1347-52; and Lu Z. Am J Cardiol. 2008 Jun 15;101(12):1689-93.

328   LI K. Heart. 2012 Jun;98(12):920-5.

CPSIA information can be obtained at www.ICGtesting.com
Printed in the USA
BVOW02s0500040815

411723BV00006B/240/P